ReadyRN

Handbook for Disaster Nursing and Emergency Preparedness

ReadyRN

Handbook for Disaster Nursing and Emergency Preparedness

SECOND EDITION

Tener Goodwin Veenema, PhD, MPH, MS, CPNP, FNAP

President and CEO
TenER Consulting Group, LLC
Associate Professor of Clinical Nursing and
Assistant Professor of Emergency Medicine
University of Rochester Medical Center
Rochester, New York

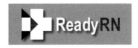

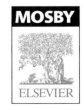

MOSBY
ELSEVIER

11830 Westline Industrial Drive
St. Louis, Missouri 63146

READYRN: HANDBOOK FOR DISASTER NURSING   ISBN: 978-0-323-06361-6
AND EMERGENCY PREPAREDNESS
Copyright © 2009 by Mosby, Inc., an imprint of Elsevier, Inc.
Copyright © 2006 by Tener Goodwin Veenema

Notice

Knowledge and best practice in this field are constantly changing. As new research and experience broaden our knowledge, changes in practice, treatment, and drug therapy may become necessary or appropriate. Readers are advised to check the most current information provided (i) on
procedures featured or (ii) by the manufacturer of each product to be administered, to verify the
recommended dose or formula, the method and duration of administration, and contraindications. It is the responsibility of practitioners, relying on their own experience and knowledge of
the patient, to make diagnoses, to determine dosages and the best treatment for each individual
patient, and to take all appropriate safety precautions. To the fullest extent of the law, neither
the Publisher nor the Author assumes any liability for any injury and/or damage to persons or
property arising out of or related to any use of the material contained in this book

The Publisher

Previous edition copyrighted 2006

Library of Congress Cataloging-in-Publication Data
Veenema, Tener Goodwin.
    ReadyRN : handbook for disaster nursing and emergency preparedness / Tener Goodwin
Veenema. -- 2nd ed.
        p. ; cm.
    Includes bibliographical references and index.
    ISBN 978-0-323-06361-6 (pbk. : alk. paper)
    1. Disaster nursing--Handbooks, manuals, etc. 2. Emergency nursing--Handbooks, manuals, etc.
I. Title. II. Title: Handbook for disaster nursing and emergency preparedness.
    [DNLM: 1. Emergencies--nursing--United States--Handbooks. 2. Disaster Planning--United
States--Handbooks. 3. Disasters--United States--Handbooks. 4. Emergency Nursing--methods--
United States--Handbooks. 5. Terrorism--United States--Handbooks. WY 49 V418r 2009]
    RT108.V44 2009
    610.73'49--dc22

                                                                            2008036566

Executive Publisher: Tom Wilhelm
Managing Editor: Maureen Iannuzzi
Senior Developmental Editor: Jennifer Ehlers
Publishing Services Manager: Jeff Patterson
Senior Project Manager: Clay S. Broeker
Design Direction: Kim Denando

Working together to grow
libraries in developing countries

www.elsevier.com | www.bookaid.org | www.sabre.org

Printed in China

ELSEVIER   BOOK AID
               International   Sabre Foundation

Last digit is the print number: 9 8 7 6 5 4 3 2 1

This book is dedicated to my husband, Ken, and my children, Kyle, Kendall, Blair, and Ryne.

Family first, last, and always. With all my love, Mom.

REVIEWERS

Margaret Irwin Crew, RN, ND
Disaster Management Consultant
Franklin, Tennessee

Cheryl K. Schmidt, PhD, RN, CNE, ANEF
Associate Professor
University of Arkansas for Medical Sciences College of Nursing
Little Rock, Arkansas

PREFACE

PURPOSE OF THE HANDBOOK

ReadyRN: Handbook for Disaster Nursing and Emergency Preparedness, second edition, has been designed for you—today's nurse. The world in which we practice today has changed dramatically, and nurses are being asked to respond to health care events for which they have had little preparation.

Hurricane Katrina in August of 2005 illustrated the health implications of the growing incidence and intensity of natural disasters. The looming threat of biological, chemical, and radiological terrorism persists. Avian and pandemic influenza appear on the global health care horizon, along with other emerging infectious diseases.

This handbook is a comprehensive yet compact resource for nurses working *in all types of health care settings.* Small and portable, it is readily accessible in a glove compartment, workbag, or purse. Designed for easy use, this handbook allows nurses to have critical information at their fingertips. The quick facts and clinical decision-making support in the handbook help nurses to respond appropriately to *any* type of disaster or public health emergency, to protect and care for their patients, and to keep themselves and their families safe.

HOW TO USE THE HANDBOOK

Keep this handbook with you or easily accessible at all times! Designed as a quick reference, this handbook is the perfect resource for emergency information and guidelines *at the point of care.* In the field, in the hospital, in the office or clinic setting, in long-term care facilities or visiting nurse sites, this handbook will help to keep you safe and prepared to respond to any major event.

Use this handbook to answer your most important questions:

- How do I keep myself safe?
- How do I care for my patients?
- Who can I call for help?
- How do I manage this event?
- Can I go home to my family?

Use this handbook as a teaching aid to better understand disaster nursing and emergency preparedness or as an on-scene reference when disaster strikes. Each chapter is divided into sections, which are outlined on the opening page of each chapter. Use these as a guide to the types of information to be found in the chapter.

Look for *Quick Q&A: Key Questions* and *Quick Answers* to the most frequently asked questions.

At the end of the handbook is a glossary of disaster nursing terms and acronyms. In addition, there are two customizable sections for each nurse to complete—a family disaster plan and a section with space to fill in local, state, and federal public health contact information.

NOTE: URLs used in this handbook are current as of the publication date.

SYMBOLS USED IN THE HANDBOOK

Many symbols are used throughout this handbook to relay critical information quickly. The symbols and their descriptions are outlined below

SYMBOL	DESCRIPTION
ANTIDOTE AVAILABLE	Antidote Available
FAMILY RISK	Family Risk—High
FAMILY RISK	Family Risk— Low
ISOLATE	Isolate Patients
ODORLESS	Odorless
PERSONAL RISK	Personal Risk—High
PERSONAL RISK	Personal Risk—Medium
PERSONAL RISK	Personal Risk—Low
QUARANTINE	Quarantine Patients
REPORTABLE DISEASE	Reportable Disease

CONTENTS

PART

1

BASICS

Disaster Management, 2

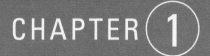

Disaster Management

CRITICAL INFO

- Appreciate the unique demands on healthcare providers during disasters and public health emergencies.
- Be prepared to fulfill your role in your agency's emergency operations plan (EOP).
- In the event of an emergency, know who is in charge, and who will be assigning job action sheets (JAS) and/or where to find them.
- Have a basic understanding of the different levels of response (local, state, and federal) and how they interact.
- Know the language of disaster communication.

QUICK Q&A

Key Question: What is different about disaster nursing than normal daily nursing practice?

Quick Answer: During a disaster event the fundamentals of good clinical nursing care remain the same. The demands of the event will alter some characteristics of nursing response, however. The focus shifts to doing the "greatest good for the greatest number with the least amount of harm." The components of practice that may change include the following:

1. Triage
2. Decontamination
3. Management: reporting will switch to an Incident Command System (ICS)
4. Allocation of scarce resources
5. Redesign/designation of facilities to accommodate surge of patients/surge capacity

OVERVIEW

Disasters are broadly defined as any destructive event that disrupts the normal functioning of the community. They may also be defined as an "occurrence, either natural or man-made, that causes human suffering and creates human needs that victims cannot alleviate without assistance" (American Red Cross, nd). Disasters have been an integral part of the human experience since the beginning of time, causing premature death, impaired quality of life, and altered health status.

Under the Robert T. Stafford Disaster Relief and Emergency Assistance Act, as amended and related authorities (FEMA 592, June 2007), *major disaster* means "any natural catastrophe (including any hurricane, tornado, storm, high water, wind-driven water, tidal wave, tsunami, earthquake, volcanic eruption, landslide, mudslide, snowstorm, or drought) or, regardless of cause, any fire, flood, or explosion, in any part of the United States, which in the determination of the President causes damage of sufficient severity and magnitude to warrant major disaster assistance under this Act to supplement the efforts and available resources of States, local governments, and disaster-relief organizations in alleviating the damage, loss, hardship, or suffering caused thereby."

Classified on the basis of their onset, duration, scope, and impact, from the standpoint of healthcare providers, the term *disasters* refers to catastrophic events that result in casualties that overwhelm the healthcare resources of the community involved.

Healthcare facilities can be affected by external or internal disasters, or both. Internal disasters occur when there is an event within the facility that poses a threat to disrupt the environment of care. External disasters become a problem for a facility when the consequences of an event create a demand for services that tax or exceed the usual available resources. External disasters may further be classified into two broad categories: natural or human-caused. See Table 1-1 for examples of external and internal disasters.

TABLE 1-1   Examples of External and Internal Disasters

EXTERNAL DISASTERS		
NATURAL	**HUMAN- CAUSED**	**INTERNAL DISASTERS**
Blizzard/extreme cold	Terrorism	Water/power/HVAC failure
Cyclone, hurricane, typhoon	• Chemical	Fire/explosion
Drought	• Biological	Flood
Earthquake	• Radiological	Loss of medical gases
Extreme heat/ heat wave	• Nuclear	Chemical/radiation release
Flooding	• Explosive	Violence/hostage-taking
Tornado	Transportation accident	Elevator emergencies
Tsunami	Industrial accident	Building collapse
Volcanic eruption	Chemical spill	Inability of staff to reach work
Wildfires		

DISASTER CHARACTERISTICS

Disasters are typically classified into two main groups: *natural disasters* and *human-caused disasters*. Understanding the differences between these two groups and their unique characteristics can help define planning and response efforts.

NATURAL DISASTERS

The World Health Organization defines a *natural disaster* as the "result of an ecological disruption or threat that exceeds the adjustment capacity of the affected community" (Lechat, 1979). Natural disasters are of many types and have diverse characteristics that will be addressed in this chapter.

HUMAN-CAUSED DISASTERS

Human-caused disasters are those events for which the principle, direct causes are identifiable human actions, deliberate or otherwise. Human-caused disasters can be divided further into three categories:

1. Complex emergencies
2. Technological disasters
3. NA-TECHS (pronounced "Nay-Teks"), or combination, disasters

Complex Emergencies

Complex emergencies involve situations where populations suffer significant casualties because of war, civil strife, or other political conflict. Some disasters are the result of a combination of forces such as drought, famine, disease, and political unrest, resulting in the displacement of millions of people from their homes.

Technological Disasters

Technological disasters are those in which large numbers of people, property, community infrastructure, and economic welfare are affected directly and adversely by any of the following:

- Major industrial accidents
- Unplanned release of nuclear energy
- Fires or explosions from hazardous substances such as fuel, chemicals, or nuclear materials

NA-TECHS

NA-TECHS occur when a natural disaster results in a secondary disaster that is the result of weaknesses in the human environment. An example of this is an earthquake triggering a chemical explosion.

Disaster Management

While most disasters can be categorized as either natural or human-caused, every disaster has a unique set of characteristics that prevents a community from developing a one-size-fits-all approach to disaster planning. "All-hazards" planning is the key to community and organizational preparedness. Understanding the impact that these disaster characteristics have on individuals and communities will be important to responding in a safe, timely, and appropriate manner.

DISASTER MANAGEMENT CONTINUUM

Each disaster is a unique event. It is important both to appreciate the characteristics of a disaster and to understand how these characteristics can vary from disaster to disaster.

Disasters are defined by the following four key characteristics:
- Onset
- Duration
- Scope
- Impact

ONSET OF A DISASTER

The *onset* of a disaster can be sudden, without warning. However, in some cases there may be minimal advance notice. Consider the timing of the following disasters and their effects:
- An earthquake that occurs late at night when everyone is asleep
- A tornado that strikes in the middle of the day when people are at work
- The detonation of a bomb during a crowded public event

DURATION OF A DISASTER

The *duration* of a disaster is measured from the time it starts (for example, when the tremors from an earthquake begin) to the time the immediate crisis has passed (when the tremors from an earthquake cease). Some disasters begin and end quite quickly, and the time from beginning to end may be seconds or minutes. Other disasters are much more prolonged (occurring over hours, days, or months), such as hurricanes, slow-rising floods, wildfires, and, in extreme cases, droughts or famine.

SCOPE OF A DISASTER

The *scope* or magnitude of a disaster involves the geographic area or region that is affected by the disaster. A disaster can be limited to a concentrated area, such as a small neighborhood or town. Alternatively, it can cover a large geographic region (e.g., the coastline communities of five states).

IMPACT OF A DISASTER

The fourth characteristic, the *impact* of the disaster, addresses more specifically the extent to which the population or community infrastructure has been affected. Disasters can strike rural areas in which very few people or community resources are impacted, or they can strike areas that are heavily populated and where the majority of a community's infrastructure may be damaged or destroyed.

All disaster response begins at the local level, and as such, communities must be prepared for whatever happens, no matter how big or small. Successful disaster response requires a community to address the following:

- Identify and anticipate disaster risks and hazards ("all-hazards").
- Prepare the material resources and skilled personnel to respond to these risks and hazards.
- Develop comprehensive plans to deploy these resources to assist the community and its recovery.
- Learn from disasters and translate the lessons learned into invaluable future preparedness.

Effective planning is the most important element of disaster management, and strong leadership is required to mobilize and focus the organization's energy. Disaster management refers to the cycle of preparing for, responding to, and recovering from a disaster. This cycle consists of the following five phases (Figure 1-1, Table 1-2, and Box 1-1):

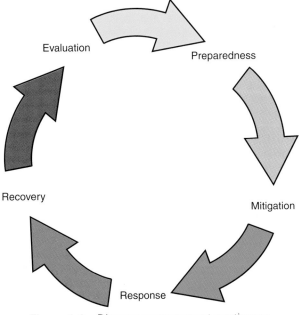

Figure 1-1. Disaster management continuum.

TABLE 1-2	The Disaster Continuum and Associated Nursing Actions		
Time	0-24 hours	24-72 hours	>72 hours
Disaster continuum	Preparedness	Response, mitigation	Recovery, evaluation
Nursing actions	Participate in development of community disaster plans	Activate local disaster response plan	Continue provision of nursing and medical care
	Participate in community risk assessment	Notification and initial response	Continue disease surveillance
	Elements of hazard analysis for "all-hazards" approach	Leadership assumes control of event	Monitor safety of food and water supply
	Hazard mapping	Command post is established	Withdraw from disaster scene
	Vulnerability analysis	Establish communications	Restore public health infrastructure
	Initiate disaster prevention measures	Conduct damage and needs' assessment at scene	Retriage and transport patients to appropriate level of care facilities
	Prevention or removal of hazard	Search, rescue, and extricate	Reunite family members
	Movement/relocation of at-risk populations	Establish field hospital and shelters	Monitor long-term physical health outcomes of survivors
	Public awareness campaigns	Triage and transport of patients	Monitor mental health status of survivors
	Establish early warning systems	Mitigate all ongoing hazards	Provide counseling and debriefing for staff
	Perform disaster drills and table-top exercises	Activate individual agency disaster plans	Provide staff with adequate time off for rest
	Identify educational and training needs for all nurses	Establish need for mutual aid relationships	Evaluate disaster nursing response actions
	Develop disaster nursing databases for notification, mobilization, and triage of emergency nurse staffing resources	Integrate state and federal resources	Revise original disaster preparedness plan
		Ongoing triage and provision of nursing care	
	Develop evaluation plans for all components of disaster nursing response	Evaluate public health needs of affected population	
		Establish safe shelter and delivery of adequate food and water supplies	
		Provide for sanitation needs and waste removal	
		Establish disease surveillance and vector control	
		Evaluate need for/activate additional nursing staff (disaster nursing response plans)	

TMTener Goodwin Veenema

BOX 1-1	The Five Phases of the Disaster Management Continuum*

1. **Preparedness** refers to the proactive planning efforts designed to structure the disaster response before its occurrence. Disaster planning assesses the risk for a given disaster to occur and evaluates its potential damage.
2. **Mitigation** attempts to limit a disaster's impact on human health and community function by taking measures to limit the amount of damage, disability, or loss of life that may occur.
3. **Response** phase is the actual implementation of the disaster plan focusing on saving lives, providing first aid, minimizing and restoring damaged systems such as communications and transportation, and providing care and basic life requirements to victims.
4. **Recovery** actions focus on stabilizing and returning the community to its preimpact status. This can range from rebuilding damaged buildings and repairing infrastructure to relocating populations and instituting mental health interventions.
5. **Evaluation** involves evaluating the response efforts to the disaster in order to better plan and prepare for future disasters.

*The Federal Emergency Management Agency (FEMA) officially recognizes only the first four phases of the disaster management continuum; however, evaluation is an important, yet frequently overlooked, phase of disaster management.

- Preparedness
- Mitigation
- Response
- Recovery
- Evaluation

ROLE OF NURSES

Nurses play a critical role in effectively coordinating and implementing any disaster response plan. They directly participate in disaster triage, transportation, and treatment of a potentially large number of victims.

Nurses may or may not have received any disaster response training before the event's occurrence. Access to disaster nursing resources and just-in-time (JIT) training programs is strongly encouraged. Nurses will also be expected to supervise unlicensed healthcare providers.

Ongoing changes in disaster healthcare policy will target new emphasis on the nation's public health infrastructure, information technology and communications' systems, immunization and antibiotic therapy guidelines, educational preparation, and numerous other aspects of daily healthcare practice. Nurses need to understand and participate in the healthcare policy development process with respect to disaster preparedness and response as planners, policy makers, educators, individuals, members of a community, and members of professional organizations. This requires knowledge of the process at the levels in which it occurs: local, state, national, and political representation at the individual as well as the organizational level.

Globalization is frequently discussed in all areas of healthcare today, including disaster relief. Nurses have been involved in international policy development through the International Council of Nurses and the World Health Organization. The direct involvement of nurses in planning for and responding to international disasters will become more important as boundaries that separate one country from another become less rigid, accessibility is improved, and the number and scope of disasters continue to increase.

LEVELS OF RESPONSE

In a disaster emergency the following three levels of response exist:
- Local
- State and regional
- Federal

LOCAL RESPONSE

All disaster responses begin at the local level. No matter the size or scale of the event, local communities are expected to provide the immediate disaster response. Local disaster response organizations include police departments, fire departments, public health departments, emergency services, and the American Red Cross (ARC). These groups protect our communities on a daily basis and may be "first to the scene" (first responders). Local hospitals (first receivers) also need to develop an emergency operations plan (EOP) for the activation of resources in the event of an internal or external disaster. The responsibilities of the hospital disaster committee include the following:
- Define what would be a disaster for the hospital.
- Review standards and guidelines developed by The Joint Commission (TJC) and local regulators addressing emergency preparedness.
- Create an EOP consistent with the Incident Command System (ICS) (discussed later in this chapter), which would allow responders to manage the command, operations, planning, logistics, and finance and administration of an incident without being hindered by jurisdictional boundaries.
- Create, review, and update the hospital plan as the institution changes, regulations are amended, or a flaw in the plan is identified.

- Assist each department with clarifying the roles of responders and predetermining leadership within the department.
- Create a uniform format for each departmental plan; include external resources for personnel, equipment, and supplies.
- Create a concise notification system to contact on-duty and off-duty personnel.
- Integrate the local, regional, and state plans into the design of the hospital plan.
- Participate in the development of the local, regional, and state disaster plans.
- Orient, educate, and reeducate all personnel to disaster activation protocols.
- Conduct and evaluate drills testing the system; amend and improve the plan.
- Critique activations of the disaster plan within the institution and community.

STATE AND REGIONAL RESPONSE

Depending on the size and type of the disaster, resources from outside the community might need to be acquired to assist in the containment and control of the incident. When state resources are requested, the state emergency management office (SEMO) will activate the state emergency operations center (EOC). The regional SEMO representative serves as the liaison between the county EOC and the state EOC and also provides the state with the necessary information to determine if and when state resources will be needed.

FEDERAL RESPONSE

There are some disasters that are so large they warrant a massive rescue and recovery response, which under most circumstances would exceed any given community's or state's resources. Under those situations, the disaster response must be raised to a national level and the state may request assistance from the federal government. The federal government response is executed under the National Incident Management System (NIMS).

The National Incident Management System

The National Incident Management System provides a consistent nation-wide template to enable federal, state, local, and tribal governments and private sector and nongovernmental organizations to work together effectively and efficiently to prepare for, prevent, respond to, and recover from domestic incidents, regardless of cause, size, or complexity, including acts of catastrophic terrorism.

The NIMS represents a core set of doctrine, concepts, principles, terminology, and organizational processes that enable effective and collaborative incident management at all levels. It is not an operational incident management or resource allocation plan. For more information about NIMS or to download the *National Incident Management System* document, refer to the Web site http://www.fema.gov/emergency/nims/index.shtm.

The National Response Framework (NRF) provides a framework for incident management at all jurisdictional levels. The framework compiles a complete spectrum of activities to include the prevention of, preparedness for, response to, and recovery from terrorism, major natural disasters, and other major emergencies. The NRF incorporates best practices and procedures from incident management disciplines—homeland security, emergency management, law enforcement, firefighting, public works, public health, responder and recovery worker health and safety, emergency medical services, and the private sector—and integrates them into a unified structure. It forms the basis of how the federal government coordinates with state, local, and tribal governments and the private sector during incidents. It establishes protocols to help accomplish the following:

- Save lives and protect the health and safety of the public, responders, and recovery workers.
- Ensure security of the homeland.
- Prevent an imminent incident, including acts of terrorism, from occurring.
- Protect and restore critical infrastructure and key resources.
- Conduct law enforcement investigations to resolve the incident, apprehend the perpetrators, and collect and preserve evidence for prosecution and/or attribution.
- Protect property and mitigate damages and impacts to individuals, communities, and the environment.
- Facilitate recovery of individuals, families, businesses, governments, and the environment.

For more information about the NRF, vist http://www.fema.gov/pdf/emergency/nrf/nrf-core.pdf.

Post Katrina Emergency Management Reform Act of 2006 (PKEMRA)

On October 4, 2006 President George W. Bush signed into law the Post Katrina Emergency Reform Act. This Act establishes new leadership positions within the Department of Homeland Security (DHS), incorporates additional functions into the Federal Emergency Management Agency (FEMA), creates and reallocates functions to other departments within the DHS, and amends the Homeland Security Act in ways that directly and indirectly affect the organization and functions of various entities within the DHS.

The Post Katrina Emergency Management Reform Act transfers, with the exception of certain offices listed in the Act, functions of the Preparedness Directorate to the new FEMA. The following entities are included in this transfer:

- The United States Fire Administration (USFA)
- The Office of Grants and Training (G&T)
- The Chemical Stockpile Emergency Preparedness Division (CSEP)
- The Radiological Emergency Preparedness Program (REPP)
- The Office of National Capital Region Coordination (NCRC)

More information about PKEMRA and its implications for federal disaster response activities can be located at http://www.dhs.gov/xabout/structure/gc_1169243598416.shtm.

Robert T. Stafford Act and the Federal Response

In 1988 the Robert T. Stafford Disaster Relief and Emergency Assistance Act was enacted to support state and local governments and their citizens when disasters overwhelm them, providing the following forms of assistance:

- Establishes a process for requesting and obtaining a *Presidential Disaster Declaration*
- Defines the type and scope of assistance available from the federal government
- Sets the conditions for obtaining that assistance

In response to Hurricane Katrina, the Act was revised and updated to the Robert T. Stafford Disaster Relief and Emergency Assistance Act, as amended and related authorities (FEMA 592, June 2007).

The *Federal Emergency Management Agency* (FEMA), now part of the Department of Homeland Security, is tasked with coordinating the national response to disaster under both the NIMS and the Stafford Act.

For more information about the Stafford Act and disaster declaration, the *Robert T. Stafford Disaster Relief and Emergency Assistance Act* is available online at http://www.fema.gov/about/stafact.shtm.

Presidential Declaration

The Stafford Act requires that all requests for a Presidential declaration be made by the governor of the affected state. The governor processes these requests through the regional FEMA/Emergency Preparedness and Response (EPR) office. State and federal officials conduct a *preliminary damage assessment* (PDA) to estimate the extent of the disaster and its impact on individuals and public facilities. This information is included in the governor's request to show that the disaster is of such severity and magnitude that an effective response is beyond the capabilities of the state and the local government and that federal assistance is necessary.

Based on the governor's request, and the supporting documentation regarding the extent of the damage, the President may declare that a major disaster or emergency exists, and activate an array of federal programs to assist in the response and recovery effort.

Federal Assistance Available under Presidential Declaration

Not all federal programs are activated for every disaster. The determination of which programs are activated is based on the needs found during the preliminary damage assessment and any subsequent information that may be discovered.

The federal assistance, coordinated by FEMA under the Emergency Preparedness Response Directorate, falls into the following three general categories:

- *Individual assistance* provides aid to individuals, families, and business owners.
- *Public assistance* provides aid to public (and certain private nonprofit) entities for certain emergency services and the repair or replacement of disaster-damaged public facilities.
- *Hazard mitigation assistance* provides funding for measures designed to reduce future losses to public and private property.

For more information, please refer to *A Guide to the Disaster Declaration Process and Federal Disaster Assistance,* which can be downloaded from http://www.fema.gov/pdf/rrr/dec_proc.pdf. Box 1-2 provides information on the distinction between an emergency and a major disaster pertaining to the Stafford Act.

BOX 1-2   Emergency vs. Major Disaster

Under the Stafford Act, the President can designate an incident either as an "emergency" or as a "major disaster." Both authorize the federal government to provide essential assistance to meet immediate threats to life and property, as well as additional disaster relief assistance.

The President may, in certain circumstances, declare an "emergency" unilaterally, but may only declare a "major disaster" at the request of a governor who certifies that the state and affected local governments are overwhelmed. Under an "emergency," assistance is limited in scope and may not exceed $5 million without Presidential approval and notification to Congress. In contrast, for a major disaster, the full complement of Stafford Act programs can be authorized, including long-term public infrastructure recovery assistance and consequence management.

DISASTER PREPAREDNESS PLANS

Several plans have been instituted to aid the different levels of emergency response. These include the following:
- National Response Framework (NRF)
- Incident Command System (ICS)
- Hospital Incident Command System (HICS)

NATIONAL RESPONSE FRAMEWORK

This plan provides a framework for how the government needs to respond to an emergency. The NRF is an "all-hazards" approach to domestic incident management and includes prevention, preparedness, response, and recovery activities. It establishes the following helpful protocols:
- Save lives and protect the health and safety of the public, responders, and recovery workers.
- Ensure security of the homeland.
- Prevent an imminent incident, including acts of terrorism, from occurring.
- Protect and restore critical infrastructure and key resources.
- Conduct law enforcement investigations to resolve the incident, apprehend the perpetrators, and collect and preserve evidence for prosecution and/or attribution.
- Protect property and mitigate damages and impacts to individuals, communities, and the environment.
- Facilitate recovery of individuals, families, businesses, governments, and the environment.
- Provide details through the 15 emergency support functions (ESFs) for the response.

The NRF is divided into 15 responsibility areas referred to as the "emergency support functions" (ESFs). Each ESF describes the responsibilities of various federal agencies for coordinating support, resources, and services to states, tribes, and other federal agencies during disasters that are nationally significant. See Table 1-3 for a listing of the 15 ESFs. For more information on the National Response Framework, visit http://www.dhs.gov/dhspublic/interapp/editorial/editorial_0566.xml.

INCIDENT COMMAND SYSTEM

The ICS pertains to disasters in the field, outside of a hospital or healthcare system. Effective coordination among local, state, and federal responders at the scene of a response is a key factor in ensuring successful responses to major incidents. In the event of a medical emergency, however, confusion and chaos are widely experienced by the hospital, staff, and first responders.

TABLE 1-3	NRP Emergency Support Functions
ESF #	**TITLE**
ESF 1	Transportation
ESF 2	Communications
ESF 3	Public Works and Engineering
ESF 4	Firefighting
ESF 5	Emergency Management
ESF 6	Mass Care, Housing, and Human Services
ESF 7	Resource Support
ESF 8	Public Health and Medical Services
ESF 9	Urban Search and Rescue
ESF 10	Oil and Hazardous Materials Response
ESF 11	Agriculture and Natural Resources
ESF 12	Energy
ESF 13	Public Safety and Security
ESF 14	Long-Term Community Recovery and Mitigation
ESF 15	External Affairs

Problems that are frequently detected in a disaster response include the following:

- Too many people reporting to one supervisor
- Different emergency response organizational structures
- Lack of reliable incident information
- Inadequate and incompatible communications
- Lack of structure for coordinated planning among agencies
- Unclear lines of authority
- Terminology differences among agencies
- Unclear or unspecified incident objectives

As a result, eight principles have been identified for adequate operation:

1. Common terminology: This minimizes confusion that may arise as a result of different terms used by different agencies.
2. Modular organization: Using a top-down approach, the incident commander will delegate duties.
3. Integrated communications: This allows the coordination of communication plans and operating procedures.
4. Unified command structure: Each person should report to one supervisor only.
5. Consolidated action plans: Follow identified goals and objectives whether verbal or written.
6. Manageable span of control: The number of individuals who report to a supervisor should be limited to five.

7. Predesignated incident facilities: Zones for areas such as decontamination, transport, and press should be clearly demarcated.
8. Comprehensive resource management: This coordinates independent resources to avoid cluttering of personnel and communications.

To minimize the confusion caused by having multiple agencies with different objectives responding to an event, the ICS was developed to allow responders to effectively manage the complexity and demands of an incident in a structured fashion without being hindered by jurisdictional boundaries. To control the communication and planning of an emergency response, the ICS divided emergency response into five functions: command, operations, planning, logistics, and finance and administration. It is vital for hospital and agency staff to be cross-trained for all of these roles to ensure that all roles can be filled in the event of personnel unavailability or injury. Each nurse's role will depend upon the specific implementation of the ICS at his/her own organization or agency.

To locate additional information about the Incident Command System, see Figure 1-2 and visit http://www.osha.gov/SLTC/etools/ics/index.html.

Hierarchy of the Incident Command System

Command staff: Responsible for all aspects of response operations. The command staff represents those positions highest on the hierarchy.
- Incident commander (IC): The mission of the IC is to organize and direct the operations of the incident. The IC establishes an EOC and then initiates a meeting to develop the initial incident action plan

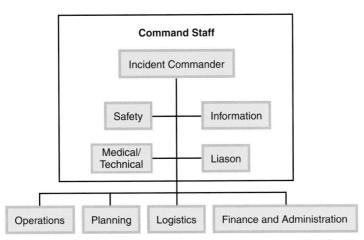

Figure 1-2.   Incident Command System structure. (From the Centers for Disease Control and Prevention.)

(IAP). The IC acts more as a "director" than a "doer" and manages on a macro level rather than a micro level.

- Safety and security officer: The mission of the safety officer is to ensure the safety of the staff, facility, and the environment during the disaster operation. The safety officer has the final authority to make decisions as they relate to safety and hazardous conditions.
- Liaison officer: The mission of the liaison officer is to function as a contact for external agencies. During times of disaster, all communication from the hospital to local, state, and federal agencies should go through the liaison officer to prevent duplicate requests or conflicting information.
- Public information officer: This position is responsible for providing information to the news media. Disaster managers must be aware that the news media can make or break the public's perception of the hospital's response to a disaster.
- Medical/technical specialist: This person provides guidance over a variety of types of events (e.g., biological, chemical, radiological, clinic administration).

General staff: Staff positions all fall under one of four sections and are headed by a chief.

1. Operations: The mission of the operations staff is to direct the actual activities related to patient care, such as medical and nursing, during disaster response.
2. Planning: The mission of the planning staff is to collect and distribute information within the organization that is required for planning and the development of an IAP.
3. Logistics: The logistics staff has a mission to ensure that all resources and support required by the other sections are readily available. It includes maintenance of the environment and procurement of supplies, equipment, and food.
4. Finance and administration: The mission of the finance staff is to monitor the utilization of assets and authorize the acquisition of resources essential for the emergency response.

HOSPITAL INCIDENT COMMAND SYSTEM (HICS)

HICS is an emergency management system that employs a logical management structure, defined responsibilities, clear reporting channels, and a common nomenclature to help unify hospitals with other emergency responders. HICS has specific disaster response role functions that are described in job action sheets (JAS) that clearly define each functional role and the tasks required to fulfill that role. The use of incident command reduces staff freelancing and provides management with the level of control necessary to manage the disaster. The HICS plan offers the following benefits:

- Predictable chain of management
- Flexible organizational chart allowing flexible response to specific emergencies
- Prioritized response checklists
- Accountability of position function
- Improved documentation for improved accountability and cost recovery
- Common language to promote communication and facilitate outside assistance
- Cost-effective emergency planning within healthcare organizations

Each nurse's role within HICS will be determined by the scope of the event and the job action sheet (JAS) that he or she is assigned.

For more information about the HICS, visit http://www.emsa.ca.gov/hics/hics.asp. An organizational chart for the HICS is shown in Figure 1-3.

NATIONAL PLANNING SCENARIOS

Scenario #1. Nuclear Detonation: 10 Kiloton Improvised Nuclear Device

Scenario #2. Biological Attack: Aerosol Anthrax

Scenario #3. Biological Disease Outbreak: Pandemic Influenza

Scenario #4. Biological Attack: Plague

Scenario #5. Chemical Attack: Blister Agent

Scenario #6. Chemical Attack: Toxic Industrial Chemicals

Scenario #7. Chemical Attack: Nerve Agent

Scenario #8. Chemical Attack: Chlorine Tank Explosion

Scenario #9. Natural Disaster: Major Earthquake

Scenario #10. Natural Disaster: Major Hurricane

Scenario #11. Radiological Attack: Radiation Dispersal Device

Scenario #12. Explosives Attack: Bombing Using Improvised Explosive Devices

Scenario #13. Biological Attack: Food Contamination

Scenario #14. Biological Attack: Foreign Animal Disease (Foot & Mouth)

Scenario #15. Cyber Attack

The national planning scenarios are broadly applicable and focus on a range of capabilities. In addition to providing the design basis for national preparedness goals and responder capability standards, the scenarios can provide the design basis for exercises throughout the nation. They have been developed in a way that allows them to be adapted to local conditions.

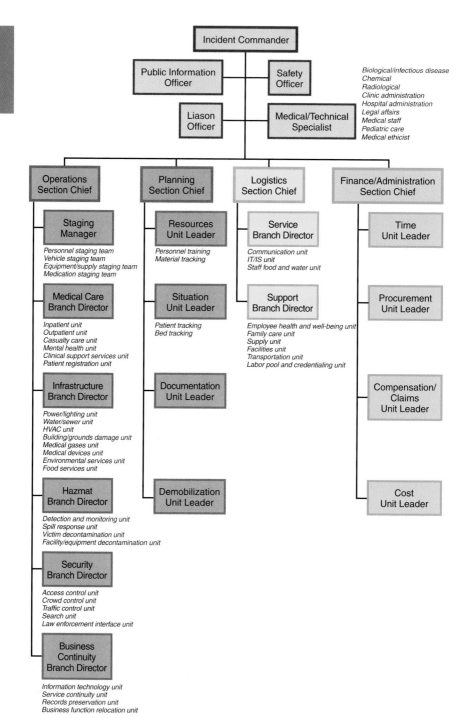

Figure 1-3. Structure of Hospital Incident Command System.

Although certain areas have special concerns—for example, continuity of government in Washington, DC; viability of financial markets in New York City; and trade and commerce in other major cities—every part of the United States is vulnerable to one or more major hazards. These scenarios should form the basis for planning for healthcare provider response as well, in light of our national preparedness goals.

Nurses need to be aware of these 15 potential disaster scenarios and BE PREPARED to participate in a response effort for any 1 of these events.

EFFECTIVE COMMUNICATION

Effective communication is vital in a disaster. To improve outcomes, nurses should be trained in the "language of disaster." A communications' plan should be developed in advance to ensure the necessary planning, preparation, and training will occur. There are eight rules to consider when devising a communications' plan:

1. Meets the needs of the user
2. Financially feasible
3. Reliable
4. Able to endure extreme environments
5. Ease of use
6. Able to work in a resource-constrained environment
7. Used regularly
8. Reviewed and updated regularly

There are three factors that affect the viability of a communications' plan:

1. Limited communication: This is typically caused by damage to the communication infrastructure, such as phone lines. This will impede the ability to contact other disaster personnel as well as state and federal governments.
2. Excessive communication: Multiple agencies may communicate conflicting information, resulting in confusion and ineffectiveness.
3. Unhelpful communication: This results from irrelevant or inappropriate communications. For example, a surge of calls from the media or worried family members may paralyze phone lines, resulting in impeded communications within the hospital.

Additionally, planning is necessary to establish alternate mechanisms in the event that a communication system is not viable. The following should be considered as potential modes of communication:

- Phone lines
- Cell phones

- E-mail and instant messaging
- Access Overload Control (for cellular radio telephones) (ACCOLC)
- Satellite
- Radio communication
- Amateur radio
- Radio and television
- Telemedicine/Internet
- "Low-tech" modes of communication, such as messengers, written information, and whiteboards

The Centers for Disease Control and Prevention (CDC) provides extensive resources to healthcare providers on emergency response communications (see http://www.bt.cdc.gov/erc/).

AMERICAN RED CROSS

MISSION

The *American Red Cross* (ARC) is a humanitarian organization of volunteers that provides relief to survivors of disasters. The Red Cross helps people prevent, prepare for, and respond to emergencies and provides such services consistent within its *Congressional Charter* and under the principles of the *International Red Cross and Red Crescent Movement.*

FUNDAMENTAL PRINCIPLES

The following are the fundamental principles of the *International Red Cross and Red Crescent Movement:*

- Humanity
- Impartiality
- Neutrality
- Independence
- Voluntary service
- Unity
- Universality

CONGRESSIONAL CHARTER

The *Congressional Charter* of 1905 states that the American Red Cross will "carry on a system of national and international relief in time of peace and apply the same in mitigating the sufferings caused by pestilence, famine, fire, floods, and other great national calamities, and to devise and carry on measures for preventing the same" (American Red Cross, nd). This Charter is not only a grant of power but also an imposition of duties and obligations to the nation, to disaster survivors, and to those donors who support its work.

Red Cross disaster relief focuses on meeting an individual's immediate disaster-caused needs. When a disaster threatens or strikes, the Red Cross provides shelter, food, and health and mental health services to address basic human needs. In addition to these services, the core of Red Cross disaster relief is the assistance given to individuals and families affected by disaster to enable them to resume their normal daily activities independently. The Red Cross also feeds emergency workers, handles inquiries from concerned family members outside the disaster area, provides blood and blood products to disaster victims, and helps those affected by disaster access other available resources.

KEY POINTS

The following are key points to remember about the American Red Cross:

- It is the result of a congressional mandate requiring action in times of emergency to alleviate human suffering.
- The ARC responds to more than 70,000 disasters nationally each year.
- The ARC receives no government funds.
- The ARC is entirely funded by the American people.
- All Red Cross assistance is free.

What is most important to remember about the role of the Red Cross in disaster relief is that the Red Cross supplements the resources and services of the local, state, and federal governments and does not override or substitute for the local, state, and federal governments' responsibilities in times of disasters.

AMERICAN RED CROSS AT THE LOCAL LEVEL

Most counties have active Red Cross chapters that meet the day-to-day needs of individuals affected by community emergencies such as single-family house fires and small floods. These needs typically include short-term shelter, food and clothing, and the provision of mental health and physical health services.

AMERICAN RED CROSS AT THE STATE AND NATIONAL LEVELS

When a disaster exceeds the human and material resources of a given Red Cross chapter, the affected chapter can look to neighboring chapters and other chapters within the state for assistance. In those situations where the incident exceeds that which the state can accommodate, the Red Cross may deploy resources from within its service area (e.g., the northeast region) or from across the country.

THE AVIATION DISASTER FAMILY ASSISTANCE ACT OF 1996

In 1996 the National Transportation Safety Board (NTSB) was assigned the role of integrating the resources of the federal government with those of local and state authorities and the airlines to meet the needs of aviation disaster victims and their families. As a result, the *Federal Family Assistance Plan for Aviation Disasters* was developed and implemented. This plan describes the airline and federal responsibilities in response to an aviation crash involving a significant number of passenger fatalities and/or injuries.

In addition, the Aviation Disaster Family Assistance Act of 1996 (ADFAA) mandates that the NTSB identify a human service organization to coordinate family assistance and mental health services to surviving victims and the families of the deceased and to coordinate a nondenominational memorial service. The NTSB, in turn, has named the American Red Cross to oversee the coordination of these services. In the event an aviation disaster meets the above criteria and the ADFAA is enacted, the national headquarters of the American Red Cross will deploy a *Critical Response Team* to engage the *Federal Family Assistance Plan for Aviation Disasters.* This team will work with local, state, and federal resources to meet the mental health and spiritual care needs of those involved.

To download the *Federal Family Assistance Plan for Aviation Disasters,* you may navigate to www.ntsb.gov/publictn/2000/spc0001.pdf. This document was prepared by the National Transportation Safety Board and published on August 1, 2000.

OTHER DISASTER RELIEF ORGANIZATIONS

During times of large-scale disasters, it is important to recognize that most communities will never have enough governmental resources to meet the immediate needs of disaster survivors. With this in mind, it is critical that a county's disaster plan include a collaboration and partnership with multiple agencies (both public and private) that can assist in meeting the needs of disaster survivors. Besides the American Red Cross, these agencies include the following:

- The Salvation Army and other faith-based organizations
- Crime victim services
- Healthcare institutions
- Business and industry

- Organizations meeting the needs of special populations (e.g., children, the physically and emotionally disabled, elders, those from various cultural and ethnic backgrounds)
- Veterinary services
- Labor unions
- Human service organizations (e.g., local community mental health centers)

For information about organizations that participate in disaster relief, consult the *National Voluntary Organizations Active in Disasters* Web site at www.nvoad.org.

For more information regarding the American Red Cross, visit the Web site at http://www.redcross.org.

NATIONAL RESPONSE FRAMEWORK

FEMA is the lead agency for implementing ESF 6 (Feeding and Sheltering) with ARC acting as the support agency for ESF 6, ESF 5 (Information and Planning), ESF 8 (Health and Medical Services), and ESF 11 (Food).

PART

2

NATURAL DISASTERS AND PUBLIC HEALTH EMERGENCIES

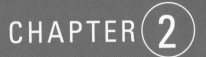

CHAPTER 2

Weather-Related and Environmental Disasters

CRITICAL INFO

- The frequency and intensity of natural disasters are increasing.
- Awareness of the types of morbidity and mortality associated with each type of natural disaster can help the nurse be better prepared to respond.
- Natural disasters result in an increased workload and unsafe environment for nurses.
- Nurses should know how to treat injuries caused by natural disasters that are prevalent in their geographic region.
- Nurses who are not trained in search and rescue should *not* enter a disaster site alone, in order to prevent becoming a disaster victim.
- Stay safe! Secure the environment before entering.
- The Federal Emergency Management Agency (FEMA) is the lead federal agency for natural disasters—you can find more information at www.fema.gov.

OVERVIEW

The World Health Organization defines a *natural disaster* as the "result of an ecological disruption or threat that exceeds the adjustment capacity of the affected community" (WHO, nd). Natural disasters occur as many different types and have diverse characteristics.

Natural disasters can be categorized as having an "acute" or "slow" onset. Examples of disasters with an acute onset include blizzards, cyclones and hurricanes, earthquakes, extreme heat waves, floods, tornadoes, tsunamis, volcanic eruptions, and wildfires; examples of disasters with slow onsets include drought. Natural disasters are unpreventable and uncontrollable; yet, they are predictable in that they occur in approximately the same geographic region. They result in long-term effects such as transportation problems and structural damage.

Natural disasters differ from environmental disasters because they are directly the result of Mother Nature, whereas environmental disasters may be human-caused. Examples of environmental disasters that can be caused either by nature or by humans include building or structural collapse, fires, food-drink poisoning, and power outage.

TYPES OF WEATHER-RELATED AND ENVIRONMENTAL DISASTERS

BLIZZARD/EXTREME COLD

A blizzard is a winter storm that is characterized by low temperatures (usually below 20° F) accompanied by high winds (at least 35 miles per hour [mph] or greater) and blowing snow that reduces visibility to a quarter mile for at least 3 hours. A severe blizzard is considered to have temperatures near or below 10° F with winds exceeding 45 mph and visibility reduced to near zero. Extreme cold is a natural disaster in which the air temperature drops to a level significantly below the usual low temperature for a specific area of the country. The exact temperature is variable, depending upon the geographic area. Because of poor visibility and hazardous road conditions, there may be an increase in motor vehicle accidents or falls.

The elderly and technology-dependent patients are particularly vulnerable during a blizzard if there is a concurrent power outage. The elderly who are without heat may require special accommodations to prevent hypothermia as well as homebound patients or patients receiving oxygen therapy. Given these considerations, surge capacity issues may arise.

Environmental Effects

- Avalanche
- Erosion
- Communication disruption
- Damage to transportation systems
- Household fires
- Snow melt and flooding
- Loss of plant/animal life
- Power/utility failures
- Heating system failure
- Healthcare system failure and overcapacity

Transportation accidents are the leading cause of death during winter storms. Preparing vehicles for the winter season and knowing how to react if stranded or lost on the road are the keys to safe winter driving. Morbidity and mortality associated with winter storms include frostbite and hypothermia, carbon monoxide (CO) poisoning, blunt trauma from falling objects, penetrating trauma from the use of mechanical snow blowers, and cardiovascular events usually associated with snow removal. Frostbite is a severe reaction to cold exposure that can permanently damage its victims. A loss of feeling and a light or pale appearance in fingers, toes, nose, or earlobes are symptoms of frostbite. Hypothermia is a condition that results when the body temperature drops to less than 90° F. Symptoms of hypothermia include uncontrollable shivering, slow speech, memory lapses, frequent stumbling, drowsiness, and exhaustion.

Nursing Implications

- Prepare to administer cardiopulmonary resuscitation (CPR) and respond to trauma injuries.
- Recognize and treat hypothermia, frostbite, falls, and miscellaneous injuries.
- Ensure safe environment for clients, adequate heat, and emergency supplies.
- Monitor protective clothing of those patients most at risk.
- Prepare to treat inhalation injuries caused by fires.
- Be aware of alternative sites with electrical power (e.g., schools, churches, hotels) in order to shelter individuals who are technology dependent.

CYCLONE, HURRICANE, AND TYPHOON

A cyclone is a large-scale storm characterized by low pressure in the center and surrounded by circular wind motion. A hurricane is a cyclone that develops in the Atlantic Ocean, while a typhoon originates in the Pacific Ocean and the China seas. Typhoon winds range from 64 to 170 mph while hurricane winds range from 74 to 175 mph. Both have five classification categories. In addition to high winds, torrential rains and storm surges can result.

Environmental Effects

- Epidemics
- Flooding
- Landslides
- Mudslides
- Erosion
- Water contamination
- Loss of plant/animal life
- Building/structural damage
- Communication disruption
- Power/utility failures
- Healthcare facility damage
- Healthcare system failure and overcapacity
- Damage to transportation systems

Nursing Implications

- Prepare to assist with timely evacuation or find shelter for affected populations.
- Prepare for traumas, injuries, and long-term illnesses from water contamination.
- Be familiar with your facility's disaster plan and any annual updates.
- Be ready to respond as soon as watches or warnings are issued.
- Social work and psychiatric referrals may be necessary.

DROUGHT

A drought is a transient, prolonged period (at least one season) of the absence of adequate precipitation that results in a shortage of water in a particular geographic area, thereby affecting the water needs of plants, animals, and humans. A drought may occur in any geographic area but may manifest in different ways. A drought may occur even when rainfall is normal but when the use of water increases or when the water supply becomes contaminated.

Environmental Effects

- Epidemics
- Erosion
- Fires
- Food/water contamination
- Loss of plant/animal life

Nursing Implications

- Prepare to treat dehydration, foodborne or waterborne illnesses, tickborne or fleaborne illnesses, and malnutrition/diseases of malnutrition.
- Have ample supplies of bottled water ready.
- Prepare to treat respiratory illnesses that may be caused by wildfires.

EARTHQUAKE

An earthquake is a sudden, rapid shaking of the earth caused by the breaking and shifting of tectonic plates under the earth's surface. Earthquakes are one of the most destructive and frightening kinds of natural disasters. They can inflict structural damage to buildings at great distances and cause other natural disasters to take place, such as flooding.

Environmental Effects

- Tsunamis
- Landslides
- Avalanches

Weather-Related and Environmental Disasters

- Flooding
- Fires
- Chemical spills
- Loss of plant/animal life
- Building/structural collapse
- Dam breaks
- Public health infrastructure failure
- Healthcare facility damage
- Damage to transportation systems
- Communication disruption
- Healthcare system failure and overcapacity

Nursing Implications

- Walking wounded will self-transport.
- Prepare for wound washing and debridement.
- Prepare to treat fractures and head injuries.
- Prepare to address the food, clothing, and shelter needs of patients.
- Prepare to care for patients with a variety of mental health effects such as severe anxiety or depression.
- Crush injuries are common in victims who are trapped and may require extrication.
- *Crush syndrome* affects many organs and is the most frequent cause of death after earthquakes, apart from trauma (Box 2-1).

Crush Injuries and Crush-Related Acute Renal Failure

Crush-related acute renal failure may occur as the result of impaired kidney perfusion and intratubular obstruction from myoglobin and uric acid accumulation. Early fluid resuscitation (within the first 6 hours, preferably BEFORE the victim is extricated) is essential. The preferred solution is

---

BOX 2-1   Major Steps in Treating Patients with Crush Syndrome

Consider the importance of early fluid administration in the field.
Closely monitor each patient's fluid intake and urinary output after admission.
Correct electrolyte abnormalities.
Remember that the healthcare team may need to consider dialysis as a life-saving procedure.

Data from Sever MS, Vanholder R, Lameire N: Management of crush-related injuries after disasters, *New Engl J Med* 354:10, 2006.

isotonic saline, given at a rate of 1 liter (L) per hour (10 to 15 milliliters [ml] per kilogram of body weight per hour), while the victim is under the rubble, followed by hypotonic saline soon after the rescue. Adding 50 milliequivalents (mEq) of sodium bicarbonate to each second or third liter of hypotonic saline (usually a total of 200 to 300 mEq the first day) will maintain a urinary pH above 6.5 and prevent the intratubular deposition of myoglobin and uric acid.

EXTREME HEAT/HEAT WAVE

Extreme heat/heat wave is a natural disaster in which there is a high level of heat and humidity that lasts for an extended duration of time. The level of heat and the duration of time of a heat wave may be variable, depending on the area of the country in which the heat wave occurs. There is marked concern for a heat wave when the daytime heat index is 105° F or higher, the nighttime temperature is 80° F or higher, and these high temperatures occur for a minimum of 48 hours.

Environmental Effects

- Drought
- Wildfires
- Erosion
- Loss of plant/animal life

Nursing Implications

- Prepare to treat heat stroke and other heat-related illnesses, such as dehydration, sunburn, heat exhaustion, heat edema, heat rash, heat cramps, heat tetany, and heat syncope.
- Cooling mechanisms should be implemented immediately.
- Rapid cooling and immediate transport to an emergency facility are indicated for all victims of heat stroke/heat syncope.
- Prepare to treat respiratory illnesses that may be caused by wildfires.
- Have oral rehydration solutions and ample supplies of bottled water, IV fluids, cooling packs, spray bottles, and fans ready to treat the signs and symptoms of dehydration.
- Prepare to treat dehydration, foodborne or waterborne illnesses, tickborne or fleaborne illnesses, and malnutrition/diseases of malnutrition.

FLOODING

A flood is a natural disaster in which there is an unusually large accumulation of water caused by one or more of the following: prolonged rainfalls, overflowing of a river or stream, or sudden ice/snow melt. Floods can also be the result of other natural disasters such as earthquakes or tsunamis. Flooding is associated with significant morbidity and mortality.

Environmental Effects

- Fire
- Epidemics
- Landslide
- Erosion
- Loss of plant/animal life
- Water/food contamination
- Building/structural collapse
- Communication disruption
- Health system failures
- Power/utility failures
- Healthcare facility damage
- Damage to transportation systems

Nursing Implications

- Prepare to treat traumatic injuries such as water intoxication, aspiration, near-drowning, crush injury, fracture, electrocution, and hypothermia.
- Prepare to treat foodborne and waterborne illnesses such as *Escherichia coli,* hepatitis A, shigellosis, vibrio and cholera, and other illnesses such as malaria caused by an increase in mosquitoes.
- Have ample supplies of bottled water ready.
- Prepare to address the food, clothing, and shelter needs of patients.
- Communities that experience flood-related disasters may have extended recovery phases and experience multiple floods, complicating recovery efforts.
- Prepare to care for patients with a variety of mental health effects such as severe anxiety or depression.

TORNADO

Tornadoes are violent, rapidly whirling air spirals that rotate a funnel of air extending from a cloud to the ground. They occur when warm, humid air meets a cold front, creating thunderstorm clouds. Tornadoes can travel for many miles at speeds of 250 mph or more and can leave behind a path of damage averaging 9 miles long by 200 yards wide.

Environmental Effects

- Flooding
- Loss of plant/animal life

- Power/utility failures
- Communication disruption
- Building/structural damage
- Healthcare facility damage
- Damage to transportation systems
- Healthcare system failure and overcapacity

Nursing Implications

- Walking wounded will self-transport.
- Prepare for wound washing and debridement.
- Prepare to treat fractures and head injuries.
- Acute stress will be exhibited by more patients after tornadoes than after other disasters.
- Prepare to address the food, clothing, and shelter needs of patients.
- Prepare to care for patients with a variety of mental health effects such as severe anxiety or depression.

TSUNAMI

A tsunami is a series of long waves generated by any rapid, large-scale shift, earthquake, landslide, volcanic eruption, or a meteorite from space. These waves can travel between 300 and 600 mph and reach heights of 100 feet or more. When a major quake is felt, the waves can reach the beach in a matter of minutes, even before a warning is issued. The largest wave is usually the fifth to the eighth to reach shore.

Environmental Effects

- Fires
- Flooding
- Epidemics
- Erosion
- Loss of plant/animal life
- Water/food contamination
- Loss of community infrastructure
- Damage to transportation systems
- Healthcare system failure and overcapacity

Nursing Implications

- Prepare for wound washing and debridement.
- Prepare to treat traumas such as fractures and head injuries.
- Prepare to address the food, clothing, and shelter needs of patients.

Weather-Related and Environmental Disasters

- Prepare to treat foodborne and waterborne illnesses such a *E. coli*, hepatitis A, shigellosis, vibrio and cholera, and other illnesses such as malaria caused by an increase in mosquitoes.
- Prepare to care for patients with a variety of mental health effects such as severe anxiety or depression.

VOLCANIC ERUPTION

A volcanic eruption is a sudden explosive eruption or flow of rock fragments and molten rock from deep inside the earth. Extreme high temperatures and pressures cause the magma beneath the earth's surface to rise, resulting in a build-up of pressure. The volcano releases the pressure by erupting. Depending on the volcano, the eruption can be minor, as in the case of Kilauea in Hawaii, or it can be violent, as in the case of Mount Pinatubo in Japan or Vesuvius in Italy.

Environmental Effects
- Wildfires
- Erosion
- Loss of plant/animal life
- Climate change
- Landslides
- Communication disruption
- Building/structural damage
- Power/utility failures
- Healthcare facility damage
- Damage to transportation systems
- Healthcare system failure and overcapacity

Nursing Implications
- Walking wounded will self-transport.
- Prepare for wound washing and debridement.
- Prepare for ash-related conditions such as respiratory problems, cardiac events, gas poisoning, and eye injuries.
- Prepare for eruption-related conditions such as orthopedic injuries, broken bones, and skin burns.
- Prepare to address the food, clothing, and shelter needs of patients.

WILDFIRES

Wildfires can be divided into three categories: surface fires, ground fires, and crown fires. A surface fire occurs most frequently and travels along the ground of the forest, destroying or killing trees. A ground fire begins when lightning strikes the forest and travels below or along the ground of the forest. Crown fires travel along the tops of the forest trees and are spread by wind.

Environmental Effects

- Flooding
- Loss of plant/animal life
- Landslides
- Mudflows
- Erosion
- Power/utility failures
- Damage to transportation systems

Nursing Implications

- Prepare to treat heat-related illnesses, such as dehydration, sunburn, heat exhaustion, heat edema, heat rash, heat cramps, heat tetany, and heat syncope.
- Watch for rhabdomyolysis and renal failure.
- Prepare to treat respiratory illnesses from smoke inhalation.
- Expect increased demand related to number of victims and bed availability with the capacity to treat burns and multiple vented patients.
- Prepare to treat foodborne and waterborne illnesses such a *E. coli,* hepatitis A, shigellosis, vibrio, and cholera caused by flooding.
- Prepare to care for patients with a variety of mental health effects such as severe anxiety or depression.

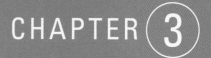

CHAPTER 3

Public Health Emergencies

CRITICAL INFO

- In the event of an environmental disaster, notify your local authorities at 911.
- The CDC Emergency Response Hotline is 1-707-488-7100.
- Public health emergencies cause a wide variety of injuries.
- They result in an increased workload and unsafe environment for nurses.
- Never enter a collapsed building unless you have had search and rescue training.
- Be aware of the potential for a secondary disaster event.

Public Health
Emergencies

OVERVIEW

An environmental disaster can be defined as an environmental emergency or ecological disruption of a severity and magnitude that results in deaths, injuries, illness, and/or property damage that cannot be effectively managed by the application of routine procedures or resources and requires additional assistance. Unlike natural disasters, environmental disasters can be the result of Mother Nature, technology, or terrorism. They are unpredictable, not limited to certain geographical boundaries, may be unpreventable in certain cases, and may cause long-term health effects. The damage environmental disasters cause is dependent on several factors: type of hazard, the mechanism of its release into the environment, the geographical location of the event, the determinants of human exposure (such as the weather conditions at the time of the event), and the length of time until the response.

TYPES OF PUBLIC HEALTH EMERGENCIES

BUILDING OR STRUCTURAL COLLAPSE

A building or structural collapse refers to the collapse of either a building or a structure. The collapse can be the result of nature, technology, human error, or terrorism.

Environmental Effects

- Power/utility failures
- Interruption of utilities
- Interruption of supplies

- Unsafe environment
- Healthcare facility failure
- Healthcare system overcapacity
- Healthcare facility overcapacity
- Healthcare facility damage
- Transportation system damage

Nursing Implications

- Walking wounded will self-transport.
- Prepare to receive patients who have required extrication.
- Prepare for wound washing and debridement.
- Prepare to treat fractures and head injuries.
- Prepare to treat crush injuries.
- Institute the emergency operations center (EOC) in your facility.
- Prepare to address the food, clothing, and shelter needs of patients.
- Prepare to care for patients with a variety of mental health effects such as severe anxiety or depression.

FIRES

A fire is caused by the combustion of flammable and inflammable materials, which produce heat, light, and smoke.

Environmental Effects

- Transportation system damage
- Interruption of utilities
- Interruption of supplies
- Unsafe environment
- Power/utility failures
- Healthcare facility or system overcapacity
- Healthcare facility failure
- Healthcare facility damage

Nursing Implications

- Prepare to treat heat-related illnesses such as dehydration, burns, heat exhaustion, heat edema, heat rash, heat cramps, heat tetany, and heat syncope.
- Watch for rhabdomyolysis and renal failure.
- Prepare to treat respiratory illnesses from smoke inhalation.
- Expect increased demand related to number of victims and bed availability with the capacity to treat burns and multiple vented patients.

- Prepare to care for patients with a variety of mental health effects such as severe anxiety or depression.
- For more information regarding burns, see Chapter 12.

FOOD-DRINK POISONING

Food-drink poisoning is an acute illness caused by ingestion of food contaminated by bacteria, bacterial toxins, viruses, natural poisons, or harmful chemical substances. It is characterized by a short incubation period (1 week or less). Infection from food-drink poisoning usually resolves itself within 1 to 2 weeks without any antibiotic treatment. Patients should, however, be rehydrated to prevent worsening of the disease.

Environmental Effects

- Panic/mass hysteria
- Epidemic

Nursing Implications

- Manage physically ill and worried well.
- Prepare to provide patients with IV hydration, antibiotics, and antiemetics.
- Prepare to treat foodborne and waterborne illnesses such as *Escherichia coli*, hepatitis A, shigella, and cholera caused by flooding.
- Prepare to provide care in absence of clean water supply.

POWER OUTAGE

A power outage is the interruption of power. It can be natural or human-caused in origin.

Environmental Effects

- Entrapment
- Health emergencies
- Transportation problems/accidents
- Power/utility failures
- Inability to conduct activities of daily living
- Motor vehicle accidents

Nursing Implications

- Prepare to handle the sudden influx of patients depending on weather conditions and length of blackout.
- Recognize and treat hypothermia and frostbite (during winter months) as well as hyperthermia and heat stroke (during summer months).

- Prepare to care for patients who come to the emergency department for routine care; provisions need to be made to move patients to areas where care can be provided.
- Prepare to treat fractures, head injuries, and crush injuries caused by motor vehicle accidents.
- Prepare to treat foodborne and waterborne illnesses such as *E. coli*, hepatitis A, shigellosis, and cholera caused by spoiled food.

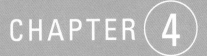

Emerging Infectious Diseases

CRITICAL INFO

- The CDC Emergency Response Hotline is 707-488-7100.
- The CDC Bioterrorism and Emerging Infectious Diseases: Bioterrorism Preparedness and Response Program number is 404-639-0385.
- Notify local public emergency responders by calling 911.
- If the infectious disease is contagious, institute appropriate isolation precautions.

QUICK Q&A

Key Question: Where do I find the most current and reliable information on pandemic or avian influenza?

Quick Answer: CDC Web page: www.cdc.gov or www.pandemicflu.gov.

OVERVIEW

Emerging and reemerging infectious diseases are classified by the Centers for Disease Control and Prevention as category C biological agents. They refer to a group of diseases either that are completely new, such as severe acute respiratory syndrome (SARS, which emerged in 2002) or that have developed new characteristics, such as multi-drug–resistant tuberculosis (MDR-TB) or extremely multi-drug–resistent tuberculosis (XDR-TB). Infectious diseases can be highly contagious and can cause widespread morbidity and mortality because of their novelty and society's lack of immunity towards them. Infectious diseases pose a significant public health threat because they can also be easily disseminated in a terrorist event.

Emerging infectious diseases (EIDs) are classified in the following three ways (Morens, Folkers, and Fauci, 2004):

1. *Emerging:* infections that have newly appeared in a population, such as SARS or avian influenza
2. *Reemerging* or *resurging:* infections that existed previously but are increasing in incidence or geographic range, such as the spread of West Nile virus and monkeypox to North America
3. *Deliberately emerging:* natural or bioengineered agents used in an act of bioterrorism, including anthrax or an agent that could be genetically modified to result in a greater impact

DIFFERENCES BETWEEN PANDEMIC INFLUENZA, ANNUAL SEASONAL INFLUENZA, AND AVIAN FLU

An influenza pandemic is a global outbreak of disease that occurs when a new influenza A virus appears or "emerges" in the human population, causes serious illness, and then spreads easily from person to person worldwide. Pandemics are different from seasonal outbreaks or "epidemics" of influenza. Seasonal outbreaks are caused by subtypes of influenza viruses that are already in existence among people, whereas pandemic outbreaks are caused by new subtypes or by subtypes that have never circulated (spread) among people or that have not circulated among people for a long time. Past influenza pandemics have led to high levels of illness, death, social disruption, and economic loss.

Usually, "avian influenza virus" refers to influenza A viruses found chiefly in birds, but infections with these viruses can occur in humans. The risk from avian influenza is generally low to most people, because the viruses do not usually infect humans. However, confirmed cases of human infection from several subtypes of avian influenza infection have been reported since 1997. Most cases of avian influenza infection in humans have resulted from contact with infected poultry (e.g., domesticated chicken, ducks, and turkeys) or surfaces contaminated with secretions/excretions from infected birds. The spread of avian influenza viruses from one ill person to another has been reported very rarely, and transmission has not been observed to continue beyond one person. Currently, concern over an outbreak of avian influenza or pandemic influenza in the United States has been increasing. As a result of antigenic shift, person-to-person transmission may result. It is widely believed that the 1918 influenza strain was originally an avian influenza.

HOW TO PROTECT YOURSELF

TRANSMISSION PRECAUTIONS

In the event of a naturally occurring infectious disease outbreak or a bioterrorist attack, additional measures may be needed to augment standard nursing precautions. Depending upon the disease, airborne, droplet, or contact precautions may be required (Table 4-1).

AIRBORNE PRECAUTIONS

Airborne transmission involves infected microorganisms or dust particles that remain suspended in the air for long periods of time and can be dispersed widely by air currents. Depending on environmental factors,

TABLE 4-1   Indicated Precautions by Diagnosis

	STANDARD	AIRBORNE	CONTACT	DROPLET
Avian influenza	X	X	X	X
Monkeypox	X	X	X	X
Nipah virus infection	X			
Norwalk-like viruses	X			
Pandemic influenza	X	X	X	X
Severe acute respiratory syndrome (SARS)	X	X	X	
Variant Creutzfeldt-Jakob disease (vCJD)	X		X	
West Nile fever	X			

a susceptible host may inhale particles within the same room or over a longer distance from the source patient. Special air handling and ventilation are required to prevent airborne transmission. In addition to standard precautions, airborne precautions include placement of the patient in a negative pressure room, use of respiratory protection such as an N95 respirator, and limitation of patient transport.

DROPLET PRECAUTIONS

Droplets can be transmitted from coughing, sneezing, and talking, and during certain procedures such as suctioning and bronchoscopy. Transmission is via the host's conjunctivae, nasal mucosa, or mouth. Droplets do not remain suspended in the air, and as such ventilation is not needed. Do not confuse with airborne transmission. In addition to standard precautions, droplet precautions include placement of the patient in a private room, use of a mask (especially when within 3 feet of the patient), and limited patient transport.

CONTACT PRECAUTIONS

Contact is the most frequent mode of transmission of nosocomial infections and is divided into direct- and indirect-contact transmission.

Direct-contact transmission involves a body-to-body contact resulting in the physical transfer of microorganisms, such as bathing or turning a patient.

Indirect-contact involves a susceptible host touching a contaminated object, such as instruments, needles, or dressings, or hands that are not washed and gloves that are not changed between patients. Gloves should always be utilized in contact precautions. Gowns should be worn if there will be body-to-body contact or the patient has diarrhea, an ostomy, or excessive wound drainage. Before leaving the room, remove gloves and gown and thoroughly wash hands; be sure to avoid contact with any contaminated surfaces.

Variant Creutzfeldt-Jakob Disease Precautions

Additional special precautions are necessary for handling and decontamination of blood, body fluids and tissues, and contaminated items from patients with confirmed or suspected variant Creutzfeldt-Jakob disease. See Variant Creutzfeldt-Jakob Disease later in this chapter, the latest College of American Pathologists (Northfield, Illinois) guidelines, or the WHO website. WHO has developed CJD infection control guidelines that can be a valuable guide to infection control personnel and other healthcare workers involved in the care of CJD patients. Destruction of heat-resistant surgical instruments that come in contact with high infectivity tissues, albeit the safest and most unambiguous method described in the WHO guidelines, may not be practical or cost effective.

QUARANTINABLE INFECTIOUS DISEASES

Federal law further stipulates that isolation and quarantine are mandated for certain communicable diseases through executive order of the President. These communicable diseases include the following:
- Cholera
- Diphtheria
- Infectious tuberculosis
- Plague
- Smallpox
- Yellow fever
- Viral hemorrhagic fevers (Lassa, Marburg, Ebola, Crimean-Congo, South American, and others)
- Severe acute respiratory syndrome
- Novel or reemergent influenza viruses that may cause a pandemic

See the following sections in Chapter 18: Isolation and Quarantine and CDC Quarantine Authority.

Emerging Infectious Diseases

EMERGING INFECTIOUS DISEASE DESCRIPTIONS

This handbook covers the following emerging infectious diseases (EIDs):
- Avian influenza (bird flu)
- Monkeypox
- Nipah virus infection
- Norwalk-like viruses
- Pandemic influenza
- Severe acute respiratory syndrome (SARS)
- Variant Creutzfeldt-Jakob disease
- West Nile fever

For information on bioterrorism agents, please see Chapter 6.
For each disease, the following information is provided:
- Diagnosis synopsis
- Weaponization
- Transmission/isolation
- Incubation, onset, and mortality
- Patient assessment/recognition
- Clinical diagnostic tests
- Patient management
- Therapy
- Personal safety risk
- Precautions
- Family safety/leaving work
- Prophylaxis/vaccine
- Public health reporting

AVIAN INFLUENZA (BIRD FLU)

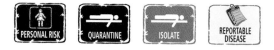

EID DESCRIPTION: AVIAN INFLUENZA (BIRD FLU)

Diagnosis Synopsis

Bird flu is an infection caused by avian influenza viruses. These flu viruses occur naturally among wild birds, which carry the viruses in their intestines. The H5N1 virus, a subtype of influenza A virus, circulates among birds worldwide and is very contagious and deadly to birds. To date, cases of wild birds and poultry with avian flu have appeared throughout Asia and have spread to birds in Europe and the Middle East.

The H5N1 virus does not usually infect humans; however, transmission from birds to people has been recorded. Most of these cases occurred from contact with infected poultry or contaminated surfaces.

Transmission of the H5N1 virus from person to person has been rare and has not continued beyond one person. However, since these viruses do not commonly infect humans, there is little or no immune protection against them in the human population. However, it is believed the virus may mutate over time, resulting in human-to-human transmission. This is referred to as "antigenic shift," which is an abrupt, major change in the virus resulting in a new subtype for which most people have little or no protection. An antigenic shift may result in a global pandemic. A vaccine for H5N1 is currently in the testing stages through the National Institute of Allergy and Infectious Diseases.

Weaponization
Aerosol inhalation.

Incubation, Onset, and Mortality
- Incubation: 2 to 3 days
- Onset: 3 days
- Mortality: 50%

Transmission/Isolation
- Transmission between persons is rare.
- Isolate patients in a negative pressure room.
- Avian influenza is a federally mandated quarantinable disease.

Patient Assessment/Recognition

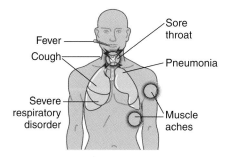

Look for typical influenza-like symptoms such as fever, cough, sore throat, and muscle aches. In addition, one or more of the following symptoms may or may not be seen: conjunctivitis, pneumonia, severe respiratory disorder, viral pneumonia, and other severe complications.

Atypical presentations of avian influenza have been reported. Patients have developed nausea, vomiting, and diarrhea preceding acute respiratory failure.

Progression to acute respiratory distress syndrome (ARDS) and respiratory failure is common. Complications have included bacterial sepsis, pulmonary hemorrhage, and multi-organ failure.

The mortality of hospitalized patients has been high because of progressive respiratory failure.

Clinical Diagnostic Tests

- Viral culture
- Immunofluorescence antibody (IFA)
- Serologic studies
- Polymerase chain reaction (PCR)

Patient Management

Patients with H5N1 should receive care in single rooms to prevent direct or indirect transmission.

Therapy

- Is resistant to amantadine and rimantadine.
- Consider oseltamivir and zanamivir when treating patients, since both are thought to be effective in treatment and prevention of avian influenza.

Personal Safety Risk

 Currently, risk is low. However, if person-to-person transmission occurs, there will be a high risk to personal safety.

Precautions

Droplet, contact, and airborne precautions.

Family Safety/Leaving Work

 Low: According to the CDC, the spread of avian influenza viruses from an ill person to another person has been reported very rarely, and transmission has not been observed to continue beyond one person. Despite low transmission risk, thorough hand washing and changing clothes before returning home are suggested.

Prophylaxis/Vaccine
None available.

Public Health Reporting
Novel influenzas, including avian influenza, are reportable to state and local health departments.

MONKEYPOX

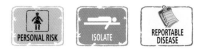

EID DESCRIPTION: MONKEYPOX

Diagnosis Synopsis
Monkeypox is a rare zoonotic orthopox virus infection that is clinically similar to smallpox. Human monkeypox primarily has been limited to the rain forest areas of central and west Africa; however, in 2003 cases were reported in Wisconsin, Illinois, and northwestern Indiana. This was the first time that cases were reported in the western hemisphere. Patients from this outbreak reported direct or close contact with infected prairie dogs. To sustain the disease in the human population, it is believed repeated animal reintroduction of monkeypox virus is needed. The disease usually lasts between 2 and 4 weeks in humans.

Weaponization
Aerosol inhalation.

Incubation, Onset, and Mortality
- Incubation: 12 days
- Onset: 1 to 3 days
- Mortality: 1% to 10%

Transmission/Isolation
- Transmitted through direct contact with the infected animal's blood, body fluids, or lesions.
- Can be spread from person to person by large respiratory droplets during direct and prolonged face-to-face contact or through direct contact with body fluids.
- Monkeypox is not as contagious as smallpox.
- Isolate patients in a negative pressure room.

Emerging Infectious Diseases

Patient Assessment/Recognition

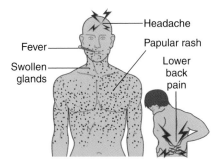

Look for fever, headache, backache, and swollen glands, as well as a papular rash covering the face, trunk, and extremities that typically progresses through stages of vesiculation, pustulation, umbilication, and crusting.

In some patients seen in the United States in 2003, early lesions became ulcerated. In addition to lesions on the head, trunk, and extremities, patients can have initial and satellite lesions on the palms, soles, and extremities. Rashes can generalize in some patients.

Clinical Diagnostic Tests

- Viral culture
- PCR
- Electron microscopy
- Immunohistochemical testing methods

Patient Management

- Therapy is primarily supportive.
- Cidofovir has been suggested as a possible treatment option in severe, life-threatening cases only.
- Patients who do require hospitalization should be placed in a negative pressure isolation room on contact, droplet, and airborne precautions; if a negative pressure room is not available, a private room should be used.

Therapy

The CDC recommends a smallpox vaccination within 2 weeks of exposure, ideally within 4 days, for exposed healthcare workers and household contacts of confirmed cases. People with weakened immune systems should not get the smallpox vaccine.

Personal Safety Risk

 Medium risk to personal safety.

Precautions

Droplet, airborne, and contact precautions.

Family Safety/Leaving Work

 Low: Minimal risk to family since monkeypox is not highly contagious.

Prophylaxis/Vaccine

Smallpox vaccine.

Public Health Reporting

Monkeypox is reportable in Massachusetts, Michigan, New York, North Carolina, and Virginia.

NIPAH VIRUS INFECTION

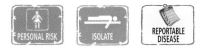

EID DESCRIPTION: NIPAH VIRUS INFECTION

Diagnosis Synopsis

Nipah virus infection is caused by a zoonotic virus belonging to the Para-myxoviridae family. It is transmitted to humans by pigs; however, cats and dogs may also become infected. The natural host of the virus is believed to be fruit bats (genus *Pteropus*), although it is not known how the bats transmit the disease to animals. The disease can have subclinical presentations where patients are asymptomatic. Nipah virus infection has only been seen in Asia and has caused a relatively mild disease in pigs in both Malaysia and Singapore. Nearly half of all survivors suffer permanent neurological sequelae.

Weaponization

Aerosol inhalation.

Incubation, Onset, and Mortality
- Incubation: 4 to 18 days
- Onset: Abrupt
- Mortality: 45%

Transmission/Isolation
- Person-to-person transmission has not been documented.
- Nipah virus was transmitted to humans, cats, and dogs through close contact with infected pigs.
- Isolate patients in a private room.

Patient Assessment/Recognition

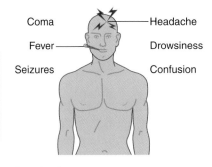

Coma — Headache

Fever — Drowsiness

Seizures — Confusion

Look for patients presenting with fever and headache lasting from 3 to 14 days, followed by drowsiness and mental confusion. The disease may progress to central nervous system (CNS) disturbances, including coma within 24 to 48 hours. Severe CNS involvement may result in death. Occasionally, respiratory tract infections have been reported during the early stages of infection.

Nipah virus can have subclinical presentations where patients are asymptomatic. Nipah virus infection has only been seen in Asia and has caused a relatively mild disease in pigs in both Malaysia and Singapore. Nearly half of all survivors suffer permanent neurological sequelae.

Clinical Diagnostic Tests
Enzyme-linked immunosorbent assay (ELISA).

Patient Management
Mechanical ventilation may be necessary.

Therapy
Therapy is supportive and symptom-specific. Therapeutic agents shorten the clinical course, prevent complications, prevent development of latency

and subsequent recurrences, decrease transmission, and eliminate established latency.

Personal Safety Risk

 Low risk to personal safety.

Precautions

Contact precautions.

Family Safety/Leaving Work

 Low: Minimal risk to family since Nipah virus is not contagious.

Prophylaxis/Vaccine

None available.

Public Health Reporting

Nipah virus infection is not a reportable disease; however, local and state public health codes typically support the reporting of unusual events that pose a public health threat.

NORWALK-LIKE VIRUSES

EID DESCRIPTION: NORWALK-LIKE VIRUSES

Diagnosis Synopsis

Noroviruses (genus *Norovirus*, family Caliciviridae) are a group of related, single-stranded RNA, non-enveloped viruses that cause acute gastroenteritis in humans. *Norovirus* was recently approved as the official genus name for the group of viruses provisionally described as "Norwalk-like viruses" (NLV). Currently, human noroviruses belong to 1 of 3 norovirus genogroups (GI, GII, or GIV), each of which is further divided into >25 genetic clusters.

Norwalk virus causes gastroenteritis. The illness is characterized by acute-onset vomiting; watery, nonbloody diarrhea with abdominal cramps; and nausea. In addition, myalgias, malaise, and headache are commonly reported. Low-grade fever is present in about half of cases. Dehydration is the most common complication and may require intravenous replacement fluids.

Weaponization
Contaminated food or water.

Incubation
The average incubation period for norovirus-associated gastroenteritis is 12 to 48 hours, with a median of approximately 33 hours.

Onset (by Exposure Type)
1 to 3 days after infection.

Duration
Symptoms usually last 24 to 60 hours. Volunteer studies suggest that up to 30% of infections may be asymptomatic.

Transmission/Isolation
Noroviruses are highly contagious, with as few as 100 virus particles thought to be sufficient to cause infection. Noroviruses are transmitted primarily through the fecal-oral route, either by direct person-to-person transmission or by fecally contaminated food or water. Noroviruses can also spread by a droplet route from vomitus. These viruses are relatively stable in the environment and can survive freezing and heating to 60° C (140° F). In healthcare facilities, transmission can additionally occur through hand transfer of the virus to the oral mucosa via contact with materials, fomites, and environmental surfaces that have been contaminated with either feces or vomitus.

Food and drinks can very easily become contaminated with norovirus because the virus is so small and because it probably takes fewer than 100 norovirus particles to make a person sick. Food can be contaminated either by direct contact with contaminated hands or work surfaces that are contaminated with stool or vomit, or by tiny droplets from nearby vomit that can travel through air to land on food. Although the virus cannot multiply outside of human bodies, once on food or in water, it can cause illness.

Some foods can be contaminated with norovirus *before* being delivered to a restaurant or store. Several outbreaks have been caused by the consumption of oysters harvested from contaminated waters. Other produce such as salads and frozen fruit may also be contaminated at source.

Typical venues for infection include the following:
• Nursing homes and residential institutions
• Restaurants and catered events
• Cruise ships

Nursing Homes and Residential Institutions

Protracted outbreaks of NLV disease have been reported among elderly persons living in institutional settings (e.g., nursing homes). In certain cases, the outbreak was initially caused by a common-source exposure to a fecally contaminated vehicle (e.g., food, water). Later, the outbreak spreads through person-to-person transmission among the residents; this spread is facilitated by the enclosed living quarters and reduced levels of personal hygiene that result from incontinence, immobility, or reduced mental alertness. Because of underlying medical conditions, the disease among these persons can be severe or fatal.

Restaurants and Catered Events

Investigations of foodborne NLV outbreaks have implicated multiple food items, including oysters, salads, sandwiches, cakes, frosting, raspberries, drinking water, and ice. Frequently, the implicated food is fecally contaminated with NLVs at its source (e.g., oysters harvested from fecally contaminated waters or raspberries irrigated with sewage-contaminated water). However, foodhandlers might contaminate food items during preparation.

Cruise Ships

Passengers and crewmembers on cruise ships and naval vessels are frequently affected by outbreaks of NLV gastroenteritis. These ships dock in countries where levels of sanitation might be inadequate, thus increasing the risk for contamination of water and food taken aboard or for having a passenger board with an active infection. After a passenger or crewmember brings the virus on board, the close living quarters on ships amplify opportunities for person-to-person transmission. Furthermore, the arrival of new and susceptible passengers every 1 or 2 weeks on affected cruise ships provides an opportunity for sustained transmission during successive cruises.

Isolation Precautions

Patients with suspected norovirus infection should be managed with standard precautions with careful attention to hand hygiene practices. However, contact precautions should be used when caring for diapered or incontinent persons, during outbreaks in a facility, and when there is the possibility of splashes that might lead to contamination of clothing. Persons cleaning areas heavily contaminated with vomitus or feces should wear surgical masks as well. In an outbreak setting, it may be prudent to place patients with suspected norovirus in private rooms or to cohort such patients.

Environmental Disinfection

There are no hospital disinfectants registered by the U.S. Environmental Protection Agency (EPA) that have specific claims for activity against noroviruses. In the absence of such products, the CDC recommends that **chlorine bleach** be applied to hard, nonporous, environmental surfaces in the event of a norovirus outbreak. A minimum concentration of 1000 parts per million (ppm) (generally a dilution 1 part household bleach solution to 50 parts water) has been demonstrated in the laboratory to be effective against surrogate viruses with properties similar to those of norovirus. Healthcare facility staff should use appropriate personal protective equipment (PPE) (e.g., gloves, goggles) when working with bleach.

Patient Assessment/Recognition

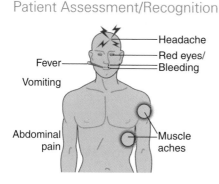

Clinical Diagnostic Tests

Look for patients presenting with acute onset of nausea, vomiting, abdominal pain, and diarrhea. Other frequently reported symptoms and signs include headache, fever, chills, and muscle aches. Pediatric patients are more likely than adults to experience vomiting, while adults are more likely to experience diarrhea.

Diagnosis of norovirus infection relies on the detection of viral RNA in the stools of affected persons, by use of reverse transcription-polymerase chain reaction (RT-PCR) assays. This technology is available at the CDC and most state public health laboratories and should be considered in the event of outbreaks of gastroenteritis in healthcare facilities. Identification of the virus can be best made from stool specimens taken within 48 to 72 hours after onset of symptoms, although good results can be obtained by using RT-PCR on samples taken as long as 7 days after symptom onset. Other methods of diagnosis, usually only available in research settings, include electron microscopy and serologic assays for a rise in titer in paired sera collected at least 3 weeks apart. Commercial enzyme-linked immunoassays are available but are of relatively low sensitivity, so their use is limited to diagnosis of the etiology of outbreaks. Because of the limited availability of timely and routine laboratory diagnostic methods, a clinical diagnosis of norovirus infection is often used, especially when other agents of gastroenteritis have been ruled out.

Patient Management

Although person-to-person spread might extend NLV gastroenteritis outbreaks, the initiating event is often the contamination of a common vehicle (e.g., food or water). Consequently, efforts to prevent both the initial contamination of the implicated vehicle and the subsequent person-to-person NLV transmission will prevent the occurrence and spread of NLV gastroenteritis outbreaks.

Therapy

The goal of therapy for viral gastroenteritis in children and adults is to prevent severe loss of fluids (dehydration). This treatment should begin at home. The CDC recommends that families with infants and young children keep a supply of oral rehydration solution (ORS) at home at all times and use the solution when diarrhea first occurs in the child. ORS is available at pharmacies without a prescription. Follow the written directions on the ORS package, and use clean or boiled water. Medications, including antibiotics (which have no effect on viruses) and other treatments, should be avoided unless specifically recommended by a physician.

Personal Safety Risk

 High risk to personal safety. Careful hand washing and infection control measures must be observed.

Precautions

- Standard and contact precautions
- Standard and contact precautions as well as surgical masks for individuals involved in cleaning the patient environment

Family Safety/Leaving Work

 Low risk to family unless direct exposure to NLV is suspected.

High risk if you suspect that you may have been infected with NLV. Avoid close contact with family members for approximately twice the incubation period.

Prophylaxis/Vaccine
None.

Public Health Reporting
Norovirus is reportable in the state of Georgia; however, local and state public health codes typically support the reporting of unusual events that pose a public health threat.

PANDEMIC INFLUENZA

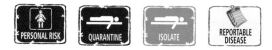

EID DESCRIPTION: PANDEMIC INFLUENZA
Diagnosis Synopsis
Influenza (flu) is a universally common epidemic illness caused by several subtypes of type A or type B influenza virus. (Type C influenza virus exists and produces a mild respiratory illness but is not believed to cause epidemics.) The most common subtypes of influenza A are H1N1 and H3N2. A new subtype of avian influenza A (H5N1) produces infrequent but often fatal human illness. (To learn more, see the previous discussion on Avian Influenza [Bird Flu].)

An influenza pandemic occurs when a new influenza A virus emerges, known as an "antigenic shift," which is an abrupt, major change in the virus resulting in a new subtype for which most people have little or no protection. A pandemic results in widespread morbidity and mortality and has serious implications for the healthcare system, including inadequate medical supplies, decreased personnel, and overwhelmed facilities. Economic and social disruptions such as travel bans and business closings would have a significant impact. Preparedness efforts should work under the assumption that the entire world population is at risk. The Spanish flu pandemic of 1918 was particularly virulent, killing more than 20 million people worldwide.

With present day biotechnology, it would be possible to produce an influenza virus weapon with traits of both the avian flu (H5N1) and the

1918 influenza viruses. As a weapon, influenza would be released as an aerosol.

Weaponization

Aerosol inhalation.

Incubation, Onset, and Mortality

- Incubation: 2 to 3 days, depending on the strain
- Onset: Abrupt, depending on the strain
- Mortality: Can be high, depending on the strain

Transmission/Isolation

- Person-to-person transmission is likely through close contact.
- Depending on the strain, the virus could be airborne.
- Patients must be isolated.
- Pandemic influenza is a federally mandated quarantinable disease.

Patient Assessment/Recognition

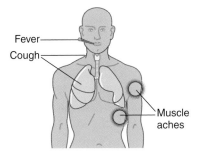

Fever
Cough
Muscle aches

Influenza presents with classic flu-like illness consisting of the sudden onset of fever, malaise, sore throat, nonproductive cough, myalgias, headache, and nasal congestion. Chills are common as are nausea and vomiting in children.

Influenza is highly contagious and is spread by aerosol droplets. The incubation period is 1 to 3 days, but it becomes contagious 1 day before the onset of symptoms. The initial symptoms produced by many of the biological weapons are nearly identical to those produced by influenza (flu-like illness). The death rate of naturally occurring influenza is low but tends to be higher in the elderly and debilitated persons. The mortality of a designer influenza containing genes from H5N1 and/or the 1918 Spanish flu would be much higher. An effective vaccine is available, but must be given annually.

When suspected, influenza can be quickly and effectively diagnosed or ruled out through the use of in-office influenza tests.

Clinical Diagnostic Tests

- Viral culture
- Immunofluorescence antibody (IFA)
- Serological studies
- PCR

Patient Management

- Isolation and quarantine are mandated by federal law.
- Isolate patients in a negative pressure room or private room.
- Administer supportive therapy of IV fluids, oxygen, and electrolytes to manage symptoms.
- Place mask on patient to prevent transmission of virus to surrounding patients and staff.

IMPORTANT NOTE: In the event of pandemic influenza, in all probability there will not be enough private or negative pressure rooms. The number of ventilators may also be limited. Sporadic shortages of basic supplies such as surgical masks may occur. It is possible that the health department will recommend that individuals remain home and shelter in place, as opposed to seeking care. It should be anticipated that a certain percent of the population will choose not to report to work (voluntary social distancing), including healthcare workers.

Therapy

- Amantadine, rimantadine, oseltamivir, and zanamivir are approved by the U.S. Food and Drug Administration for the treatment and/or prevention of influenza.
- New strains of influenza viruses may be resistant to antibiotics.

Personal Safety Risk

 High risk to personal safety.

Precautions

Airborne, contact, and droplet precautions.

Family Safety/Leaving Work

 High risk to family: Pandemic influenza is highly contagious. If you suspect that you may have been infected with the influenza virus, avoid close contact with family members for approximately twice the incubation period.

Prophylaxis/Vaccine

A vaccine probably would not be available in the early stages of a pandemic because scientists must first develop a vaccine specific for the emergent strain. It probably will take several months for a vaccine to be widely available.

Public Health Reporting

Influenza is reportable in the following states: Arkansas, Colorado, Delaware, District of Columbia, Georgia, Hawaii, Maine, Massachusetts, Michigan, Minnesota, Missouri, Montana, Nebraska, Nevada, New Mexico, New York, North Dakota, Ohio, Pennsylvania, South Carolina, South Dakota, Tennessee, Utah, Vermont, Virginia, West Virginia, and Wyoming. However, most local and state public health codes typically support the reporting of unusual events that pose a public health threat.

SEVERE ACUTE RESPIRATORY SYNDROME

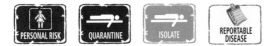

Emerging Infectious Diseases

EID DESCRIPTION: SEVERE ACUTE RESPIRATORY SYNDROME

Diagnosis Synopsis

Severe acute respiratory syndrome (SARS) is a viral respiratory illness caused by a coronavirus known as SARS-associated coronavirus (SARS-CoV). SARS was first reported in Asia in February 2003, and over a short time, the illness spread to more than 2 dozen countries in North America, Europe, and Asia before being contained. According to the World Health Organization (WHO), a total of 8098 people worldwide became sick with SARS and 774 died (WHO, nd). In the United States, eight people had laboratory evidence of SARS-CoV infection, and all of these people had traveled to other parts of the world with SARS. SARS proved to be most fatal in children, the elderly, and those with underlying chronic diseases.

Weaponization

Aerosol inhalation.

Incubation, Onset, and Mortality

- Incubation: 2 to 7 days
- Onset: 2 days
- Mortality: <10%

Transmission/Isolation

- Close contact is required.
- Patients must be isolated in a negative pressure room.
- SARS is a federally mandated quarantinable disease.

Patient Assessment/Recognition

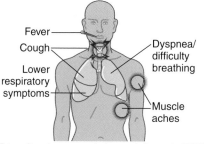

History of travel or exposure to documented/suspected SARS

Look for patients presenting with fever, shortness of breath, cough, and pneumonia. There may be a prodromal illness consisting of fever, myalgias, headaches, and diarrhea. The respiratory phase starts 2 to 7 days after the prodrome with a dry cough and mild dyspnea. The spectrum of the illness can vary from a mild variant to a rapid and severe respiratory decline with hypoxia and features of ARDS. Among hospitalized patients, 10% to 20% eventually require mechanical ventilatory support. The physical examination findings may be mild and disproportionate to the chest x-ray findings. A petechial rash may be seen. Peripheral blood lymphocytopenia and thrombocytopenia are common. The liver enzymes creatine kinase and serum lactate dehydrogenase can have elevated levels. There may be signs of disseminated intravascular coagulation. Acute renal failure has been reported.

Clinical Diagnostic Tests

- Chest radiograph
- Pulse oximetry
- Complete blood count with differential
- Blood cultures
- Sputum Gram stain and culture
- Testing for viral respiratory pathogens, notably influenza A and B and respiratory syncytial virus
- Legionella and pneumococcal urinary antigen testing
- RT-PCR testing

Medical Management

- Isolation and quarantine are mandated by federal law.
- Isolate patients in a negative pressure room.
- The management of patients with SARS is largely supportive.

Therapy

No known therapy exists. The CDC highly recommends that patients suspected or confirmed as having SARS receive the same treatment that would be administered if they had any serious community-acquired pneumonia.

Personal Safety Risk

 High risk to personal safety. **IMPORTANT NOTE:** During the SARS outbreak in Toronto, Canada, healthcare providers were disproportionately represented in the infected group. Use of contact and airborne precautions is critical to the prevention of transmission of this disease.

Precautions

Contact and airborne precautions.

Family Safety/Leaving Work

 High: SARS is highly contagious. If you suspect that you may have been infected with SARS, avoid close contact with family members for approximately twice the incubation period.

Prophylaxis/Vaccine

None available.

Public Health Reporting

Report suspected SARS cases to local and state public health agencies.

Emerging Infectious Diseases

VARIANT CREUTZFELDT-JAKOB DISEASE

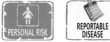

EID DESCRIPTION: VARIANT CREUTZFELDT-JAKOB DISEASE

Diagnosis Synopsis

The variant form of Creutzfeldt-Jakob disease (vCJD) is related to bovine spongiform encephalopathy (BSE), "mad cow disease," but should not be confused with the classic form of Creutzfeldt-Jakob disease (CJD) that is endemic throughout the world. Variant CJD has different symptoms and different epidemiology, and affects a younger population than does the classic form of CJD. The median age at death for vCJD patients is 28 years, compared with 68 years for patients with classic CJD. The median duration of illness for vCJD is 14 months, compared to 5 months for classic CJD. vCJD is a human prion disease that causes a neurodegenerative disorder. The clinical presentation of prominent psychiatric symptoms and delayed neurological signs, the progressive nature of the disease, and the failure to find any other diagnoses are the hallmarks of vCJD. This disease is fatal.

Weaponization

Contamination of meat products.

Incubation, Onset, and Mortality

- Incubation: 4 to 5 years for CJD; unknown for vCJD
- Onset: 4 to 5 months for CJD; 13 to 14 months for vCJD
- Mortality: 100% for CJD; 100% for vCJD

Transmission/Isolation

- Transmitted by consuming contaminated meat products.
- No person-to-person transmission occurs.
- Isolation is not necessary.

Patient Assessment/Recognition

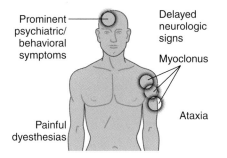

Patients present with prominent psychiatric or sensory symptoms and delayed onset of neurological abnormalities, including ataxia within weeks or months, dementia and myoclonus late in the illness, a duration of illness of at least 6 months, and a diffusely abnormal nondiagnostic electroencephalogram.

vCJD can only be confirmed through examination of brain tissue obtained by biopsy or at autopsy.

Patient Management

Supportive therapy.

Therapy

No specific therapy has been shown to stop the progression of vCJD. Therefore treatment is supportive.

Personal Safety Risk

 Low risk to personal safety.

Precautions

Standard precautions.

Family Safety/Leaving Work

 Low: No risk to family since vCJD is not contagious.

Prophylaxis/Vaccine

None available.

Public Health Reporting

Creutzfeldt-Jakob Disease is reportable in the following states: Arkansas, Connecticut, Mississippi, Nebraska, Ohio, Rhode Island, Texas, Utah, Vermont, Virginia, and Wyoming.

WEST NILE FEVER

EID DESCRIPTION: WEST NILE FEVER

Diagnosis Synopsis

West Nile fever (WNF) is caused by infection with a virus of the genus *Flavivirus*. The vector of transmission is the *Culex, Aedes,* and *Mansonia* mosquitoes as well as some ticks, with birds as intermediate hosts. The virus is endemic in several temperate climates around the world including North America, Europe, Africa, and Australia. Most cases in these regions occur during the late summer and fall.

Occasionally an associated hepatitis or encephalitis can be life-threatening. Fever and severe frontal headache, backache, and anorexia may precede the CNS signs and symptoms of encephalitis, for which the mortality rate is 40%. Mild illnesses usually resolve in less than 1 week, but prolonged fatigue is common.

Weaponization

Aerosol inhalation.

Incubation, Onset, and Mortality

- Incubation: 3 to 14 days
- Onset: within 2 weeks
- Mortality: 3% to 15%

Transmission/Isolation

- Transmission occurs via a mosquito vector.
- There is no person-to-person transmission.
- Isolation is not necessary.

Patient Assessment/Recognition

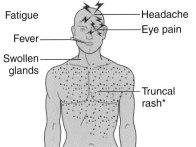

Fatigue
Fever
Swollen glands
Headache
Eye pain
Truncal rash*

*Rash presents in only 50% of cases

Most cases are asymptomatic. Patients usually present with mild illness of fever, headache, fatigue, and myalgias, and an occasionally associated macular and papular rash on the upper body. The rash is typically viral exanthem resembling measles (morbilliform) or roseola.

Occasionally an associated hepatitis or encephalitis can be life-threatening. The incubation period is typically 3 to 14 days. Fever and severe frontal headache, backache, and anorexia may precede the CNS signs and symptoms of encephalitis (confusion, neck stiffness, cranial nerve palsies, and generalized weakness), for which the mortality rate is 40%.

Mild illnesses usually resolve in less than 1 week, but prolonged fatigue is common. Symptoms of encephalitis may persist for weeks or may be permanent.

Clinical Diagnostic Tests

- IgM antibody-capture enzyme-linked immunosorbent assay (MAC-ELISA)
- Plaque-reduction neutralization test (PRNT)
- PCR

Patient Management

Supportive therapy of IV fluids and electrolytes.

Therapy

Supportive therapy with intravenous fluids and electrolytes, assisted respiration as indicated, and anticonvulsants are the mainstays of treatment.

Personal Safety Risk

 Low risk to personal safety.

Emerging Infectious Diseases

Precautions

Standard precautions.

Family Safety/Leaving Work

 Low: Minimal risk to family since West Nile Fever is not contagious.

Prophylaxis/Vaccine

None available.

PART

3

WEAPONRY AND HUMAN-CAUSED DISASTERS

Chemical Emergencies

CRITICAL INFO

- Notify local emergency responders by calling 911.
- Call Poison Control Center at 1-800-222-1222.
- Call Centers for Disease Control Emergency Response hotline at 1-770-488-7100.
- Do not wait for test results to begin immediate treatment.
- Wear proper protective equipment when handling hazardous materials and when treating exposed patients.

QUICK Q&A

Key Question: Should I purchase a gas mask?

Quick Answer: No. A mask would only protect you if you were wearing it at the exact moment a chemical attack occurred.

To work effectively, masks must be specially fitted to the wearer, and wearers must be trained in their use. This is usually done for the military and for workers in industries and laboratories who face routine exposure to chemicals and germs on the job. Gas masks purchased at an Army surplus store or off the Internet carry no guarantees that they will work. Also, masks are manufactured to be fitted with a specific cartridge or filter that is made to work with a specific chemical or related group of chemicals. So, unless you know the chemical to which you are being exposed and you have a fresh cartridge or filter for that chemical, there is nothing else in the air to worry about. Gas masks will not protect one from a hypoxic environment!

In brief, no guarantees whatsoever are provided. More serious is the fact that the masks can be dangerous. There are reports of accidental suffocation when people have worn masks incorrectly, as happened to some Israeli civilians during the Persian Gulf War.

Chemical Emergencies

QUICK COMPARISONS

As a result of their toxic, explosive, and flammable properties, chemicals continue to be the weapons of choice for terrorist attacks. A variety of toxic chemicals may be used as chemical warfare agents. These may be categorized as shown in Table 5-1.

The onset of symptoms may not always be immediate; sometimes they may be delayed by several hours, as is the case with certain vesicants and pulmonary agents (Table 5-2). Exposure to these agents can cause serious injury and death, and thus rapid detection of the chemical is critical to the

TABLE 5-1   Chemical Agent Descriptions and Examples

AGENT CATEGORY	BRIEF DESCRIPTION	EXAMPLE
Nerve agents	Most toxic of known chemical warfare agents; nerve agents inhibit body's normal functions	Sarin
Biotoxins	Poisonous substances produced by living organisms	Ricin
Vesicants	Chemical agents that cause blisters or sores	Mustard gas
Tissue (blood) agents	Tissue (blood) agents cause chemical asphyxiation by preventing body tissues from utilizing oxygen	Cyanide
Pulmonary agents	Chemicals that cause severe irritation or swelling of respiratory tract	Chlorine
Riot control agents	Chemical compounds that temporarily inhibit person's ability to function by causing irritation to eyes, mouth, throat, lungs, and skin (i.e., tear gas)	Chlorobenzyl-idenemalo-nonitrile

TABLE 5-2   Chemical Agent Initial Symptoms and Signs

AGENT CATEGORY	RESPIRATORY	NEURO-LOGICAL	SKIN/EYES	OTHER
Nerve	Gasping Bronchocon-striction	Seizures Twitching	Tearing Eye irritation Blurred vision	Drooling Sweating Muscle weakness
Biotoxin (aerosolized ricin)	Cough Dyspnea Chest pain			Nausea Fever
Vesicants	Coughing Severe respiratory irritation		Itching Burning Blistering	
Tissue (blood)	Hyperventilation, shortness of breath	Dizziness Convulsions Loss of con-sciousness	Flushing	Nausea
Pulmonary	Coughing Runny nose Throat irritation Dyspnea Pulmonary edema	Headache	Tearing Eye irritation and pain Blurred vision	
Riot control	Chest tightness Cough		Eye irritation Tearing	

protection of first responders and emergency medical personnel, as well as to the effective treatment of victims.

CHEMICAL AGENTS: HOW TO PROTECT YOURSELF

At the scene, nurses should not be first responders, unless they are trained members of a hazardous materials (Hazmat) or fire response team. Nurses should remain outside the response zones to avoid becoming a victim. Table 5-3 refers to nurses working as first receivers at the hospital.

CHEMICAL AGENT DESCRIPTIONS

The following sections discuss each agent category in more detail. For each agent category, the following information is provided:
- Overview
- Recognition
- Exposure route(s) and associated onset of symptoms
- Duration and mortality
- Patient assessment
- Clinical diagnostic tests
- Patient management
- Therapy (includes information on antidotes if available)
- Personal safety risk
- Precautions
- PPE
- Family safety
- Public health reporting

NERVE AGENTS

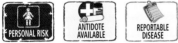

CHEMICAL AGENT DESCRIPTION: NERVE AGENTS

OVERVIEW

Nerve agents are highly toxic compounds that inhibit the body's normal functions. They are the most toxic of the known chemical warfare agents, which makes them a danger to humans and potential weapons in the hands of terrorists.

Nerve agents can be dispersed as aerosols/vapors or liquids. Nerve agent vapors are readily absorbed by inhalation and ocular contact and result in

TABLE 5-3   Protection against Chemical Agents

AGENT CATEGORY	RESPIRATORY PROTECTION	SKIN/OCULAR PROTECTION
Nerve	Pressure-demand SCBA or wall-mounted air supply or PAPR with appropriate cartridge for that chemical	• Chemical-protective clothing • Butyl rubber gloves • Chemical goggles and face shield
Biotoxin (aerosolized ricin)		• Tychem BR or Responder CSM chemical-protective clothing • Full face-piece respirator provides eye protection • Personal protective equipment
Vesicants		• Butyl rubber chemical protective gloves • Chemical goggles and face shield
Tissue (blood) agents		*Arsine/phosphine:* Chemical-protective clothing is not generally required because arsine gas is not absorbed through skin and does not cause skin irritation. However, contact with the liquid (compressed gas) can cause frostbite injury to skin or eyes. *Cyanides:* Chemical-protective clothing is recommended because both hydrogen cyanide vapor and liquid can be absorbed through skin to produce systemic toxicity. Face shield or eye protection should also be worn.
Pulmonary	Pressure-demand SCBA or wall-mounted air supply or PAPR with appropriate cartridge for that chemical	• Chemical-protective clothing • Chemical goggles and face shield *Phosphides:* Chemical-protective clothing is not generally required because phosphine gas is not absorbed through skin and skin irritation is unlikely. Use rubber gloves and aprons with victims exposed to phosphides.
Riot control		• Chemical-protective clothing is not generally required • Eye protection may be necessary to avoid eye irritation

immediate local and systemic effects. The liquid form of the agent is also readily absorbed through the skin.

Nerve agents are divided into two categories: G agents and V agents. Examples of both follow:

- *G agents:* sarin (GB), soman (GD), tabun (GA)
- *V agents:* VX

RECOGNIZING NERVE AGENTS

Table 5-4 shows how to recognize nerve agents by appearance and odor.

EXPOSURE TYPES AND ONSETS

Table 5-5 indicates the onset of symptoms for each type of possible exposure.

DURATION AND MORTALITY

Recovery may take several months. Permanent damage to the central nervous system is possible after exposure to a high dose. G agents are lethal within 1 to 10 minutes and V agents are generally lethal within 4 to 18 hours, depending on dose and route of entry.

TABLE 5-4	Nerve Agents by Appearance and Odor	
AGENT	**APPEARANCE**	**ODOR**
Sarin	Clear, colorless	Odorless
Soman	Clear, colorless	Slight camphor odor (e.g., Vicks Vapo-Rub) or rotting fruit odor
Tabun	Clear, colorless	Faint fruity odor
VX	Clear, amber-colored	Odorless

TABLE 5-5	Nerve Agent Exposure Types and Onsets
EXPOSURE	**ONSET**
Inhalation	Immediate onset of symptoms
Ingestion	Readily absorbed
Skin/eye	Onset depends on concentration; can be delayed by several hours

PATIENT ASSESSMENT

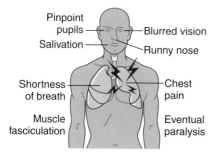

Pinpoint pupils
Blurred vision
Salivation
Runny nose
Shortness of breath
Chest pain
Muscle fasciculation
Eventual paralysis

Muscle fasciculations and eventual paralysis may occur. Symptoms usually occur within seconds of exposure to a nerve agent but may take several hours when exposure is only transdermal.

Effects and time of onset of a nerve agent are dependent upon the concentration of the agent and the amount of time exposed, as well as the route of exposure.

- *Mild inhalational exposure:* rapid onset of miosis, blurry vision, runny nose, chest tightness, dyspnea, and possible wheezing.
- *Severe inhalational exposure:* sudden coma, seizures, flaccid paralysis with apnea, miosis, diarrhea, and a victim who is "wet" (lacrimation, salivation, urination, sweating, copious upper and lower respiratory tract secretions).
- *Mild dermal exposure:* sweating and muscle fasciculations localized to the area of exposure, nausea, vomiting, diarrhea, and possible miosis.
- *Severe dermal exposure:* sudden coma, seizures, flaccid paralysis with apnea, miosis, diarrhea, and a victim who is "wet" (lacrimation, salivation, urination, sweating, copious upper and lower respiratory tract secretions). Onset of symptoms may be delayed by 30 minutes following exposure as the agents transit the skin.

Victims of a terrorist attack will usually have both inhalational and dermal exposures. Hours after treatment/decontamination, the agent, still in transit through the skin, may produce sudden and severe symptoms.

CLINICAL DIAGNOSTIC TESTS
Red blood cell or serum cholinesterase level.

PATIENT MANAGEMENT
- Do not approach contaminated victims unless wearing proper personal protective equipment.
- Supportive therapy and assisted ventilation as needed.

THERAPY

 Antidote: atropine and pralidoxime. Additional treatment (Table 5-6) would include benzodiazepines for seizures (not true antidote).

PERSONAL SAFETY RISK

 High, because of off-gassing vapor. However, if the patient is fully decontaminated, the risk is low.

PRECAUTIONS

- Maximum: standard, airborne, droplet, and contact precautions.
- Nerve agents are rapidly absorbed through the skin and may cause systemic toxicity.

PPE

See Table 5-7 for recommended PPE for nerve agents.

Chemical Emergencies

TABLE 5-6	Nerve Agent Treatment by Exposure Type
EXPOSURE	**TREATMENT**
Inhalation	• If severe signs, immediately administer, in rapid succession, all three nerve agent antidote kit(s), Mark I* injectors (or atropine if directed by physician).
	• If signs and symptoms are progressing, use injectors at 5-20 minute intervals; use no more than three injections.
	• Give artificial respiration if breathing has stopped or is difficult; do not use mouth-to-mouth if face is contaminated.
Skin	• Decontaminate using soap and water.
Eyes	• Immediately flush eyes with water for 10-15 minutes.
	• Don respiratory protective mask.
Ingestion	• Do not induce vomiting.
	• Immediately administer nerve agent antidote kit, Mark I.*

Source: CDC at http://www.bt.cdc.gov/chemical/.
*Mark I kits contain atropine 2 mg and 2-PAMCI 600 mg in separate auto-injectors.

TABLE 5-7	Recommended PPE for Nerve Agents
PROTECTION	**DESCRIPTION**
Respiratory	Pressure-demand SCBA is recommended in response situations that involve exposure to any nerve agent vapor or liquid. However, at a hospital as a first RECEIVER only PAPR WITH APPROPRIATE filter is OK.
Skin/ocular	Chemical-protective clothing and butyl rubber gloves are recommended when skin contact is possible because nerve agent liquid is rapidly absorbed through skin and may cause systemic toxicity. Wear chemical goggles and face shield.

FAMILY SAFETY

 Low: Shower and change clothes before going home.

NERVE AGENTS IN CHILDREN: GUIDELINES

See Table 5-8 for treatment guidelines for children exposed to nerve agents.

BIOTOXINS (RICIN)

CHEMICAL AGENT DESCRIPTION: BIOTOXINS (RICIN)

OVERVIEW

Ricin is derived from the castor bean *(Ricin communis)* and can be ingested, injected, or aerosolized for inhalation. Ricin is less toxic than some other biological agents but is very stable. A similar agent, abrin (derived from rosary peas) is about 25 times more toxic, but less common. Intoxication occasionally occurs in children who ingest castor beans or rosary peas.

The CDC has designated ricin as a category B bioterrorism agent. Ricin was developed as a biological weapon by the United States and its allies during World War II. Extracting the toxin is relatively easy, and Iraq and several terrorist groups are known to have produced ricin. A terrorist attack would be by aerosol release. The mortality rate of ricin is variable and

TABLE 5-8	Nerve Agents in Children			
SYMPTOMS	TRIAGE LEVEL: DISPOSITION	ATROPINE (CORRECT HYPOXIA BEFORE IV USE [RISK OF TORSADES, VFib])	PRALIDOXIME	DIAZEPAM MAY USE OTHER BENZODIAZEPINES (e.g., MIDAZOLAM)
Asymptomatic	Delayed: observe	None	None	None
Miosis, mild rhinorrhea	Delayed: admit or observe prn	None	None	None
Miosis and any other symptom	Immediate to moderate: admit	0.05 mg/kg IV or IM Repeat as needed q5-10min until respiratory status improves	25-50 mg/kg IV or IM; may repeat every hour Watch for: Muscle rigidity Laryngospasm Tachycardia	For any neurological effect: 30 days to 5 years: 0.05-0.3 mg/kg IV to max of 5 mg/dose 5 years and older: 0.05-0.3 mg/kg IV to max of 10 mg/dose May repeat q15-30min
Apnea, convulsions, cardiopulmonary arrest	Immediate to severe: admit intensive care status	0.05-0.1 mg/kg IV, IM, per ETT No maximum Repeat q5-10min as above	25-50 mg/kg IV or IM as above	See above

largely route specific. Mortality from ricin poisoning can be high depending on the dose and route of exposure.

HOW YOU COULD BE EXPOSED TO RICIN

- It would take a deliberate act to make ricin and use it to poison people—accidental exposure to ricin is highly unlikely, but happens when people eat/chew castor beans!
- People can inhale ricin mist or powder and be poisoned.
- Ricin can also get into water or food and then be swallowed.
- Pellets of ricin, or ricin dissolved in a liquid, can be injected into the body.
- Depending on the route of exposure (such as injection or inhalation), as little as 500 micrograms of ricin could be enough to kill an adult. A 500-microgram dose of ricin would be about the size of the head of a pin. If the ricin were ingested, however, a greater amount would likely be needed to cause death.

RECOGNIZING BIOTOXINS

Table 5-9 shows how to identify ricin by appearance and odor.

EXPOSURE TYPES AND ONSETS

Table 5-10 indicates the onset of symptoms for each type of possible exposure.

DURATION AND MORTALITY

Death from ricin poisoning could take place within 36 to 72 hours of exposure, depending on the route of exposure and the dose received. If death has not occurred in 3 to 5 days, the victim usually recovers.

Chemical Emergencies

TABLE 5-9	Identifying Biotoxins by Appearance and Odor	
BIOTOXIN	**APPEARANCE**	**ODOR**
Ricin	Liquid, crystalline, dry powder	Odorless

TABLE 5-10	Biotoxin (Ricin) Exposure Types and Onsets
EXPOSURE	**ONSET**
Inhalation	Within 8 hours
Ingestion	Less than 6 hours
Skin/eye	Within 8 hours

PATIENT ASSESSMENT

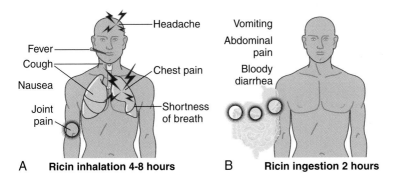

A   **Ricin inhalation 4-8 hours**   B   **Ricin ingestion 2 hours**

- *Ricin inhalation:* The initial symptoms of ricin poisoning begin 4 to 8 hours after inhalation and include fever, nausea, cough, dyspnea, chest pain, and arthralgias. Ricin poisoning may progress to pulmonary edema, acute respiratory distress syndrome (ARDS), and cyanosis. A lethal dose would result in death within 36 to 72 hours.
- *Ricin ingestion:* Symptoms begin within 2 hours of ingestion and include abdominal pain, nausea, vomiting, and gastrointestinal (GI) hemorrhaging with bloody vomit and diarrhea. The condition may progress to liver, spleen, and kidney failure and death.

CLINICAL DIAGNOSTIC TESTS
Enzyme-linked immunosorbent assay (ELISA) using respiratory tract secretions, serum, and direct tissue.

PATIENT MANAGEMENT
Supportive therapy for multiple system organ failure.

THERAPY
There is no antidote for ricin poisoning.

HOW RICIN POISONING IS TREATED
Because no antidote exists for ricin, the most important factor is avoiding ricin exposure in the first place. If exposure cannot be avoided, the most important action is then getting the ricin off or out of the body as quickly as possible. Ricin poisoning is treated by providing victims supportive medical care to minimize the effects of the poisoning. The types of supportive medical care would depend on several factors, such as the route by which victims were poisoned (that is, whether poisoning was by inhalation, ingestion, or skin or eye exposure). Care could include such

Chemical Emergencies

measures as helping victims breathe, giving intravenous medications/ fluids, administering medications to treat conditions such as seizures and low blood pressure, flushing stomachs with activated charcoal (if the ricin has been very recently ingested, within 1 hour), or rinsing victims' eyes with water if their eyes are irritated (Table 5-11).

PERSONAL SAFETY RISK

 Low: Individuals not present where the ricin was found are unlikely to have been exposed to levels high enough to negatively affect their health.

PRECAUTIONS

Standard precautions.

PPE

See Table 5-12 for PPE for biotoxins.

TABLE 5-11	Biotoxin (Ricin) Treatment by Exposure Type
EXPOSURE	**TREATMENT**
Inhalation	• Provide fresh air, rest. • Assume half-upright position. • If breathing is difficult, administer oxygen. • Perform CPR if necessary.
Skin	• Remove contaminated clothes. • Rinse skin with plenty of water (and soap if available) or shower.
Eyes	• Immediately flush with large amounts of tepid water for at least 15 minutes.
Ingestion	• May be fatal—however, the death rate even among symptomatic patients is generally low. • Do not induce vomiting. Rinse mouth. Use slurry of activated charcoal if ingestion within 1 hour. If individual is drowsy or unconscious, do not give anything by mouth. In event of vomiting, lean patient forward or place on left side (head-down position, if possible) to maintain open airway and prevent aspiration. • Early and aggressive IV fluid and electrolyte replacement required.

Chemical
Emergencies

TABLE 5-12	Recommended PPE for Biotoxins
PROTECTION	**DESCRIPTION**
Respiratory	Pressure-demand, SCBA is recommended in response situations that involve exposure to ricin in a form that may be inhaled.
Skin/ocular	Tychem BR or Responder CSM chemical-protective clothing is recommended or regular chemical PPE. Full face-piece respirator provides eye protection.

FAMILY SAFETY

 Low: Remove clothing, shower, and dispose of your clothing before going home.

VESICANTS

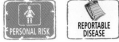

CHEMICAL AGENT DESCRIPTION: VESICANTS

OVERVIEW

Vesicants are chemical agents that produce vesicles on the skin. Vesicants include mustards, lewisites, and phosgene oxime (Table 5-13). Vesicants or "blister agents" were the most commonly used chemical warfare agents during World War I. Out of the vesicants, mustard has been used the most frequently and has been responsible for 80% of chemical-related casualties.

The most likely routes of exposure are inhalation, dermal contact, and eye contact. Ingestion of the chemical is also possible; however, it is rare. Upon inhalation of the highly reactive compound, vesicants combine with proteins, DNA, and other cellular components to result in cellular changes immediately after exposure.

RECOGNIZING VESICANTS

Table 5-14 shows how to identify vesicants by appearance and odor.

Chemical
Emergencies

TABLE 5-13   Examples of Vesicants

MUSTARDS	LEWISITES	OTHER
Distilled mustard (HD)	Lewisite	Phosgene oxime (CX)
Mustard gas (H)	(L, L-1, L-2, L-3)	
Mustard/lewisite (HL)	Mustard/lewisite (HL)	
Mustard/T		
Nitrogen mustard		
(HN-1, HN-2, HN-3)		
Sesqui mustard		
Sulfur mustard (H)		

TABLE 5-14   Identifying Vesicants by Appearance and Odor

VESICANT	APPEARANCE	ODOR
Nitrogen mustard	Colorless to yellow	Fishy, musty, soapy, or fruity
Sulfur mustard	Yellow or brown	Garlic, onions, or mustard
		NOTE: Sometimes has no odor
Lewisite	Colorless	Geraniums
Phosgene oxime	Colorless	Irritating odor

EXPOSURE TYPES AND ONSETS

Table 5-15 indicates the onset of symptoms for each type of possible exposure.

DURATION AND MORTALITY

The severity of the illness is dependent on the amount and route of exposure to the vesicant, the type of vesicant, and the medical condition of the person exposed. Exposure to high concentrations may be fatal.

PATIENT ASSESSMENT

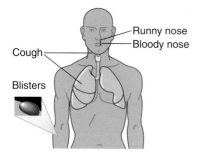

Runny nose
Bloody nose
Cough
Blisters

TABLE 5-15	Vesicant Exposure Types and Onsets	
AGENT	**EXPOSURE**	**ONSET**
Nitrogen mustard	Inhalation	Several hours
	Ingestion	Several hours
	Skin/eye	6-12 hours
Sulfur mustard	Inhalation	Several hours
	Ingestion	Several hours
	Skin/eye	4-8 hours
Lewisite	Inhalation	Rapid
	Ingestion	15-20 minutes
	Skin/eye	15-30 minutes
Phosgene oxime	Inhalation	Immediate
	Ingestion	No human data
	Skin/eye	Immediate

All of these vesicant agents act by producing direct irritation and have similar clinical presentations.

- *Ocular:* redness and burning of the eyes with lacrimation, blepharospasm, and lid edema.
- *Upper airway:* nasal irritation and discharge, sinus burning, nosebleeds, sore throat, cough, and laryngitis.
- *Pulmonary:* dyspnea, necrosis of large airway mucosa with sloughing, chemical pneumonitis, pulmonary edema, ARDS, respiratory failure.
- *Skin:* irritation and redness with delayed production of wheals, vesicles, or bullae, followed later by areas of necrosis.

See Table 5-16 for assessment tips for specific vesicants.

CLINICAL DIAGNOSTIC TESTS

- Complete blood count (CBC)
- Glucose
- Serum electrolytes
- Chest x-ray
- Pulse oximetry (or arterial blood gas [ABG] measurements)

PATIENT MANAGEMENT

- Decontaminate patients before treating.
- Provide supportive therapy.

THERAPY

There is no antidote. See Table 5-17 for treatments.

Chemical
Emergencies

TABLE 5-16   Agent-Specific Tips for Assessment

AGENT	ASSESSMENT TIPS
Sulfur mustard	Vesicles will have "string of pearls" appearance and will then coalesce Hoarse voice or barking cough typically present or aphonia if victim is exposed to high concentration
Lewisite	Single vesicle in erythematous area
Phosgene oxime	Areas of dermal blanching with an erythematous ring within 30 seconds of exposure, progressing to a wheal within 30 minutes Tissue necrosis after about 24 hours; NO vesicle!

TABLE 5-17   Vesicant Treatment by Exposure Type

EXPOSURE	TREATMENT
Inhalation	• Move patient to fresh air. • Administer oxygen and assist ventilation as required.
Skin	• Remove contaminated clothing. • Decontaminate by using soap and water or 0.5% hypochlorite solution.
Eyes	• Immediately flush eyes with water for 10-15 minutes.
Ingestion	• Do not induce vomiting. Rinse mouth. • If vomiting occurs, lean patient forward or place on left side (head-down position, if possible) to maintain open airway and prevent aspiration.

PERSONAL SAFETY RISK

 Low risk to personal safety.

PRECAUTIONS

Standard precautions.

PPE

See Table 5-18 for appropriate PPE for vesicants.

FAMILY SAFETY

 Low: Remove clothing, shower, and dispose of your clothing before going home.

TABLE 5-18	Recommended PPE for Vesicants

PROTECTION	DESCRIPTION
Respiratory	• Pressure-demand, SCBA is recommended in response situations that involve exposure to any level of lewisite and mustard-lewisite mixture vapor, or PAPR with appropriate filter in a first receiver scenario.
Skin/ocular	• Personal protective equipment and butyl rubber chemical protective gloves are recommended at all times when these chemicals are suspected to be involved. • Chemical goggles and face shield should also be worn.

TISSUE (BLOOD) AGENTS

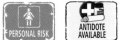

CHEMICAL AGENT DESCRIPTION: TISSUE (BLOOD) AGENTS

Chemical Emergencies

OVERVIEW
Tissue (blood) agents are poisons that affect the body by being absorbed into the blood. With the exception of arsine, tissue (blood) agents can be dispersed as liquids, aerosols, and gases that may be inhaled, ingested, or absorbed through skin and/or eye contact.

Examples of tissue (blood) agents are as follows:
• Arsine (SA) and phosphine
• Carbon monoxide
• Sodium monofluoroacetate (compound 1080)
• Cyanides
Cyanogen chloride
Hydrogen cyanide
Potassium cyanide
Sodium cyanide

RECOGNIZING TISSUE (BLOOD) AGENTS
See Table 5-19 for information on identifying tissue (blood) agents.

EXPOSURE TYPES AND ONSETS
Table 5-20 shows exposure types and onsets for tissue (blood) agents.

TABLE 5-19   Identifying Tissue (Blood) Agents by Appearance and Odor

AGENT	APPEARANCE	ODOR
Arsine	Colorless	Mild garlic or fishy
Carbon monoxide	Colorless	Odorless
Cyanides	Colorless or pale-blue	Bitter almond

TABLE 5-20   Tissue (Blood) Agent Exposure Types and Onsets

AGENT	EXPOSURE	ONSET
Arsine	Inhalation	Within several hours
Carbon monoxide	Inhalation	Minutes to hours
Cyanides	Inhalation	Seconds to minutes
	Skin/eye	30-60 minutes
	Ingestion	Rapidly fatal
Sodium monofluoroacetate	Inhalation	Minutes to hours

TABLE 5-21   Mortality of Tissue (Blood) Agents

AGENT	MORTALITY
Arsine	Highly toxic; severely exposed people are unlikely to survive
Cyanide	Patients with supportive therapy and antidotes can survive

DURATION AND MORTALITY

See Table 5-21 for mortality of tissue (blood) agents.

PATIENT ASSESSMENT

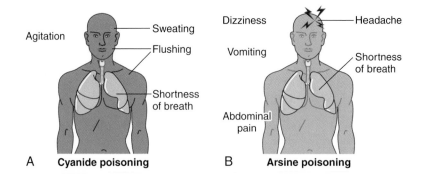

A   Cyanide poisoning

B   Arsine poisoning

- *Cyanide poisoning:* The latency period for cyanides ranges from 10 to 15 seconds up to several minutes. The signs and symptoms of mild cyanide poisoning are nonspecific and may be difficult to differentiate from other chemical warfare agents. The signs and symptoms of moderate to severe cyanide poisoning are profound and may appear similar to those of the nerve agents. Cyanogen chloride is an irritant and may produce lacrimation and upper airway irritation. When exposed to low concentrations of the other three forms of cyanide, victims will have 10 to 15 seconds of gasping, tachypnea, tachycardia, flushing, sweating, headache, giddiness, and dizziness, followed by nausea, vomiting, agitation, and confusion. At higher concentrations, the victim will have all the previously mentioned initial signs and symptoms, followed by bradycardia, apnea, seizures, shock, coma, and death. In all cases, death is caused by respiratory arrest and can be prevented by cardiopulmonary resuscitation (CPR). Cyanosis is a rare finding. Pupils may be unresponsive and dilated, but this is not specific to cyanide poisoning.
- *Arsine/phosphine poisoning:* Upon inhalation there may be a burning sensation in the chest followed by chest pain, but there may be no symptoms at all, leaving the victim unaware that he/she has been exposed. The length of time between exposure and exhibiting symptoms depends upon the concentration and duration of exposure. A delay of 2 to 24 hours is typical before the onset of any symptoms. Initial symptoms of arsine poisoning include nausea, vomiting, headache, malaise, weakness, dizziness, abdominal pain, dyspnea, and, occasionally, red-stained conjunctivae. Symptoms progress to include hematuria, jaundice, and possibly renal failure. A slight odor of garlic may be detectable on the breath. Urine may appear bloody, and patients may experience numbness, tingling, burning or prickling, memory loss, and disorientation. Severe anemia, low blood pressure, and an elevated serum potassium level may be caused by hemolysis 2 to 24 hours after exposure. Later, look for enlargement of the liver, yellowing of the skin and whites of the eyes, or a bronze appearance to the skin. Approximately 2 to 3 weeks after exposure to arsine, Mees' lines (horizontal white lines of the nails) may be observed.

CLINICAL DIAGNOSTIC TESTS
- CBC
- Blood glucose
- Electrolyte determinations

Chemical Emergencies

PATIENT MANAGEMENT

Closely monitor serum electrolytes, calcium, blood urea nitrogen (BUN), creatinine, hemoglobin, and hematocrit measurements. For victims of arsine poisoning, avoid high levels of fluid replacement as congestive heart failure (CHF) may result.

THERAPY

- *Cyanide poisoning:* Contrary to popular belief, the effects of cyanide poisoning are not irreversibly fatal, and victims may be successfully resuscitated by proper circulatory and respiratory support until the antidote can be administered.

- Cyanide antidote: amyl nitrite perles (not routinely used because there is minimal benefit); however, two other items in kit are VERY useful: sodium nitrite and sodium thiosulfate. *Instructions:* Break perle onto gauze pad and hold under nose or place under the lip of oxygen mask. Inhale for 30 seconds every minute and use a new perle every 4 minutes if sodium nitrate infusions are delayed. The literature suggests limited data on its usefulness. Consider sodium nitrate and thiosulfate.

- *Arsine/phosphine poisoning:* There is no antidote for arsine or phosphine poisoning. Do **not** administer arsenic chelating drugs. See Table 5-22 for more information on tissue (blood) agent treatment.

PERSONAL SAFETY RISK

 Low risk to personal safety.

PRECAUTIONS

Standard precautions.

PPE

Table 5-23 shows appropriate PPE for tissue (blood) agents.

FAMILY SAFETY

 Low: Minimal risk to family; remove any wet or possibly contaminated clothing before going home.

TABLE 5-22	Blood Agent Treatment by Exposure Type
EXPOSURE	**TREATMENT**

Inhalation	• Respiratory symptoms: administer supplemental oxygen by mask.
	• If patient has bronchospasms: treat with aerosolized bronchodilators or cardiac sensitizing agents. (Arsine poisoning is not known to pose additional risk during use of bronchial or cardiac sensitizing agents.)
	• Children with stridor: administer racemic epinephrine aerosol.
	  • Dose: 0.25-0.75 ml of 2.25% racemic epinephrine solution in 2.5 ml of water.
	  • Repeat every 20 minutes as needed, cautioning for myocardial variability.
	• If hemolysis develops: initiate urinary alkalinization.
	• Add 50-100 mEq of sodium bicarbonate to 1 L of 5% dextrose in 0.25% normal saline and administer IV at a rate that maintains urine output at 2-3 ml/kg/hour; maintain alkaline urine (i.e., pH >7.5) until urine is hemoglobin free.
	• If anemia develops as a result of hemolysis, consider blood transfusions.
	• Renal failure: consider hemodialysis.

Skin	• Irrigate with lukewarm (42° C) water.
Eyes	• Thoroughly irrigate with lukewarm (42° C) water or saline. • Examine eyes for corneal damage and treat appropriately.

Chemical Emergencies

PULMONARY AGENTS

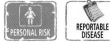

PERSONAL RISK   REPORTABLE DISEASE

CHEMICAL AGENT DESCRIPTION: PULMONARY AGENTS

OVERVIEW

Pulmonary agents (also referred to as choking or lung agents) are chemicals that cause severe irritation or swelling of the respiratory tract.

They are all liquids and gases, but they cause the most damage by being inhaled. These agents cause toxic poisoning by entering the lungs and disrupting the alveolar-capillary membrane. The misbalance that occurs

TABLE 5-23	Recommended PPE for Tissue (Blood) Agents

BLOOD AGENT	PROTECTION	DESCRIPTION
Cyanides	Respiratory	Positive-pressure, SCBA and full face-piece respirators are recommended in response situations that involve exposure to potentially unsafe levels of hydrogen cyanide.
	Skin/ocular	Chemical-protective clothing is recommended because both hydrogen cyanide vapor and liquid can be absorbed through skin to produce systemic toxicity. Chemical goggles and face shield should also be worn.
Arsine and phosphine	Respiratory	Positive-pressure, SCBA and full face-piece respirators are recommended.
	Skin/ocular	Chemical-protective clothing is generally not required because arsine gas is not absorbed through skin and does not cause skin irritation. However, chemical-protective clothing should be worn if arsine is in liquid form (compressed gas) since contact with liquid can cause frostbite injury to skin. Chemical goggles and face shield should be worn if arsine is in liquid form since contact with liquid can cause frostbite injury to eyes. *Exception:* Phosphides: Chemical-protective clothing is not generally required because phosphine gas is not absorbed through skin and skin irritation is unlikely. Use rubber gloves and aprons with victims exposed to phosphides.

reduces oxygen exchange and allows fluid to leak into the interstitial tissues and alveoli. Cutaneous contact can result in frostbite or a burn. The following are considered to be pulmonary agents:

- Ammonia
- Bromine
- Chlorine

- Hydrogen chloride
- Methyl bromide
- Methyl isocyanate
- Osmium tetroxide
- Phosgene/diphosgene
- Phosphorus (elemental, white or yellow)
- Sulfuryl fluoride

RECOGNIZING PULMONARY AGENTS

Table 5-24 shows how to identify pulmonary agents by appearance and odor.

EXPOSURE TYPE(S)/ONSET

Exposure by inhalation, ingestion, or skin/eye contact leads to immediate onset of symptoms, which may be delayed by as much as 48 hours.

DURATION AND MORTALITY

The duration and risk of mortality depend on the amount of exposure and the patient's physical characteristics.

Chemical Emergencies

TABLE 5-24	Identifying Pulmonary Agents by Appearance and Odor	

PULMONARY AGENT	APPEARANCE	ODOR
Ammonia	Colorless	Bleach
Bromine	Brownish	Bleach
Chlorine	Yellow-green	Pungent, irritating
Hydrogen chloride	Colorless, yellowish	Pungent
Methyl bromide	Colorless	Odorless or fruity/floral/sweet
Methyl isocyanate	Colorless	Pungent
Osmium tetroxide	Colorless, pale yellow	Pungent, chlorine-like
Phosgene	Colorless or white to pale yellow cloud	Pleasant odor of newly mown hay or green corn
Phosphorus	"Smoking" or "luminescent"	Garlic
Sulfuryl fluoride	Colorless	Odorless

PATIENT ASSESSMENT

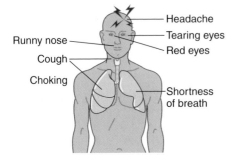

Initial symptoms include eye pain, redness, and lacrimation; sore throat; runny nose; coughing; and headache.

After hours to several days, victims may develop nausea, hemoptysis, and the signs and symptoms of pulmonary edema including choking, dyspnea, rales, hemoconcentration, hypotension, and possible cyanosis. Hypoxia and hypotension within 4 hours of exposure carries a poor prognosis.

Rarely, depending upon concentration/time, pulmonary edema can occur within 30 minutes to 4 hours for chlorine and between 2 and 6 hours for phosgene. Most fatalities are within the first 24 hours because of respiratory failure.

CLINICAL DIAGNOSTIC TESTS
- CBC
- Glucose determinations
- Electrolyte determinations
- Chest radiography
- Pulse oximetry (if severe inhalation exposure is suspected)

PATIENT MANAGEMENT
- Provide supportive therapy.
- Monitor blood pH if chlorine poisoning is suspected.

THERAPY/ANTIDOTE
No antidote is available. See Table 5-25 for treatments.

PERSONAL SAFETY RISK

  Low risk to personal safety.

TABLE 5-25   Pulmonary Agent Treatment by Exposure Type

EXPOSURE	TREATMENT

Inhalation	• Respiratory symptoms: administer supplemental oxygen by mask.
	• If patient has bronchospasms: treat with aerosolized bronchodilators or cardiac sensitizing agents.
	• Children with stridor: administer racemic epinephrine aerosol.
	  • Dose: 0.25-0.75 ml of 2.25% racemic epinephrine solution in 2.5 ml of water.
	  • Repeat every 20 minutes as needed, cautioning for myocardial variability.
	• Observe patients carefully for 6-12 hours for signs of upper airway obstruction.
	• Patients who have had a severe exposure may develop noncardiogenic pulmonary edema.

Skin	• Treat chemical burns like thermal burns. • If victim has frostbite, treat by rewarming affected areas in water bath at temperature of 102-108° F (40-42° C) for 20-30 minutes and continue until a flush has returned to affected area.
Eyes	• Continue irrigation for at least 15 minutes or until pH of conjunctival fluid has returned to normal. • Test visual acuity. • Examine eyes for corneal damage and treat appropriately.
Ingestion	• Do not induce vomiting. • Do not administer activated charcoal. • Do not perform gastric lavage or attempt neutralization after ingestion. • If not given during decontamination, give 4-8 ounces of water by mouth to dilute stomach contents. • Consider endoscopy to evaluate extent of gastrointestinal tract injury.

Chemical Emergencies

PRECAUTIONS

Standard precautions. **NOTE:** Gas or liquid pulmonary agents are caustic and corrosive and cause irritation and chemical burns upon contact with the eyes, skin, respiratory tract, or alimentary canal.

PPE

• *Respiratory protection:* Positive-pressure, self-contained breathing apparatus (SCBA) is recommended in response situations that involve exposure to potentially unsafe levels of ammonia. For a hospital setting or any first receiver setting, an appropriate respirator, including a powered air purifying respirator (PAPR) with appropriate filter, is acceptable.

- *Skin/ocular protection:* Chemical-protective clothing is recommended because pulmonary agents can cause skin irritation and burns. Face shield or eye protection should also be worn.

FAMILY SAFETY/LEAVING WORK

 Low: Decontamination is usually not needed. Remove any contaminated clothing.

RIOT CONTROL AGENTS

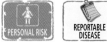

CHEMICAL AGENT DESCRIPTION: RIOT CONTROL AGENTS

OVERVIEW

Riot control agents are chemical compounds that temporarily inhibit a person's ability to function by causing irritation to the eyes, mouth, throat, lungs, and skin. Sometimes known as "tear gas," riot agents are present in both liquid and solid form and can be released in the air as fine droplets or particles.

Several different compounds are considered to be riot control agents. The three major agents are as follows:

- Chloroacetophenone (CN), also known as mace
- Chlorobenzylidenemalononitrile (CS)
- Diphenylaminearsine (DM)

RECOGNIZING RIOT CONTROL AGENTS

See Table 5-26 for information on identifying riot control agents.

EXPOSURE TYPE(S)/ONSET

Exposure to riot control agents by inhalation or by contact with the skin and/or eyes leads to rapid onset of symptoms.

DURATION AND MORTALITY

The situation will improve 15 to 30 minutes after the exposure ends. Death can be immediate when serious chemical burns are present in the throat and lungs.

TABLE 5-26	Identifying Riot Control Agents by Appearance and Odor	
RIOT CONTROL AGENT	**APPEARANCE**	**ODOR**
CN (chloroacetophenone)	White	Fragrant (e.g., apple blossoms)
CS (chlorobenzylidene-malononitrile)	White	Pungent (e.g., pepper)
DM (diphenylaminearsine)	Yellow-green	Odorless

PATIENT ASSESSMENT

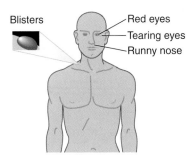

Riot control agents primarily affect the eyes, causing temporary blindness because of lacrimation and blepharospasm. They also produce conjunctival redness; cough; chest tightness; sneezing; and mouth, nose, and throat irritation. In raw or abraded skin, lacrimators can cause burning and erythema. Rarely, under conditions of high temperature, high humidity, and high concentration, vesicles may form hours later on exposed skin areas.

CLINICAL DIAGNOSTIC TESTS

No laboratory tests.

PATIENT MANAGEMENT

No specific treatment is required. The situation improves within 30 minutes after the exposure ends.

THERAPY/ANTIDOTE

No antidote is available. Table 5-27 describes treatment options.

PERSONAL SAFETY RISK

 Low risk to personal safety.

TABLE 5-27	Riot Control Agent Treatment by Exposure Type

EXPOSURE	TREATMENT
Inhalation	• Get more oxygen into patient's blood. • Use bronchodilators and steroids to help patients breathe.
Skin	• Use standard burn management techniques, including medicated bandages.
Eyes	• Immediately flush eyes with saline or water for 10-15 minutes.

PRECAUTIONS

Standard precautions.

PPE

- *Respiratory protection:* Positive-pressure, self-contained breathing apparatus is recommended in response situations that involve exposure to potentially unsafe levels of hydrogen cyanide.
- *Skin/ocular protection:* Chemical-protective clothing is not generally required. Eye protection may be necessary to avoid eye irritation.

FAMILY SAFETY/LEAVING WORK

Low: Remove any contaminated clothing. Shower before going home.

SOURCES FOR MORE UPDATED INFORMATION

- United States Army Medical Research Institue of Chemical Defense (USAMRICD): http://chemdef.apgea.army.mil
- Centers for Disease Control and Prevention (CDC): http://www.cdc.gov
- Agency for Toxic Substances and Disease Registry (ATSDR): http://www.atsdr.cdc.gov
- American College of Medical Toxicology located at http://www.acmt.net
- American Association of Poison Control Centers (AAPCC): http://www.aapcc.org/DNN
- *OSHA Best Practices for Hospital-Based First Receivers of Victims from Mass Casualty Incidents Involving the Release of Hazardous Substances:* http://www.osha.gov/dts/osta/bestpractices/html/hospital_first receivers.html

Biological Agents

CRITICAL INFO

- The CDC Emergency Response hotline is 1-707-488-7100.
- Notify local public emergency responders by calling 911.
- If you suspect a possible biological agent, begin treatment immediately; do not wait for test results.
- If the biological agent is contagious, institute appropriate isolation precautions.

QUICK Q&A

Key Question: Should I get my own supply of antibiotics?

Quick Answer: As nurses know, there are a number of different germs a bioterrorist or, for that matter, Mother Nature might use to carry out a biological attack or naturally occurring infectious disease outbreak. Many antibiotics are effective for a variety of diseases, but there remains no antibiotic that is effective against all diseases. Thus no single pill can protect against all types of biological weapon attacks. Keeping a supply of antibiotics on hand poses other problems because the antibiotics have a limited "shelf life" before they lose their strength.

There is currently no justification for "stockpiling" or taking antibiotics. Also, it should be known that antibiotics can cause side effects. They should only be taken with medical supervision.

HOW TO PROTECT YOURSELF

Bioterrorism can be defined as the intentional release or threatened release of disease-producing living organisms or biologically active substances derived from organisms and intended to cause death, illness, incapacity, economic damage, or fear. Many different types of biological agents exist, including bacteria, viruses, fungi, genetically altered or enhanced infectious agents, vaccine-resistant and/or multi–drug-resistant organisms, and toxins that are produced from organisms but resemble chemical agents. One of the main functions of these agents is to incite fear and panic, overwhelm medical and social services, disable the economy, and cause widespread morbidity and mortality.

CLASSIFICATION OF BIOLOGICAL AGENTS

The Centers for Disease Control and Prevention categorizes biological agents according to characteristics such as accessibility, ease of use, and

TABLE 6-1	Categories of Biological Agents
CHARACTERISTICS	**DISEASES**
Category A • Easily disseminated or transmitted from person to person • Result in high death rates and have potential for major public health impact • Cause public panic and social disruption • Require special action for public health preparedness	• Anthrax • Botulism • Plague • Smallpox • Tularemia • Viral hemorrhagic fevers
Category B • Moderately easy to disseminate • Result in moderate morbidity rates and low death rates • Require specific enhancements of CDC's diagnostic capacity and enhanced disease surveillance	• Brucellosis • Food/water safety threats • Glanders • Melioidosis • Psittacosis • Q fever • Ricin toxin • Staphylococcal enterotoxin B • Typhus • Viral encephalitis

Category C
• Emerging infectious diseases that could be engineered for mass dissemination because of their:
  • Availability
  • Ease of production and dissemination
  • Potential for high morbidity and death rates and major health impact
	• Nipah virus
	• Hantavirus
	• Monkeypox
	• Severe acute respiratory syndrome (SARS)
	• vCJD
	• Avian influenza
	• Pandemic flu

Biological Agents

potential for causing a public health burden. The categories are labeled as A, B, and C (Table 6-1).

ISOLATION AND QUARANTINE

Federal law stipulates that isolation and quarantine are mandated for the following diseases caused by biological agents:

- Cholera
- Diphtheria
- Infectious tuberculosis
- Plague
- Smallpox
- Yellow fever

- Viral hemorrhagic fevers (Lassa, Marburg, Ebola, Crimean-Congo, South American, and others)
- Severe acute respiratory syndrome (SARS)
- Novel or re-emergent influenza viruses that may cause a pandemic

TRANSMISSION PRECAUTIONS

In the event of a bioterrorist attack, additional measures may be needed to augment standard nursing precautions (Table 6-2). Depending upon the agent, airborne, droplet, or contact precautions may be required.

Airborne Precautions

Airborne transmission involves infected microorganisms or dust particles that remain suspended in the air for long periods of time and can be dispersed widely by air currents. Depending on environmental factors,

TABLE 6-2 Indicated Precautions by Diagnosis*	STANDARD	AIRBORNE	CONTACT	DROPLET
Anthrax, inhalational	X			
Botulism	X			
Brucellosis	X		X	
Cholera	X			
Crimean-Congo	X	X	X	X
Ebola	X	X	X	X
E. coli	X		X	
Glanders	X		X	X
Hantavirus	X			
Lassa	X		X	X
Marburg	X	X	X	X
Melioidosis	X		X	
Plague	X			
Psittacosis	X			X
Q fever	X			
Ricin toxin	X			
Salmonellosis	X			
Shigellosis	X		X	
Smallpox	X	X	X	
Staphylococcal enterotoxin B	X			
Tularemia	X			
Typhus, epidemic	X		X	
Viral encephalitides	X			

*For some VHFs, transmission patterns are not clear and all precautions should be exercised.

a susceptible host may inhale particles within the same room or over a longer distance from the source patient. Special air handling and ventilation are required to prevent airborne transmission. In addition to standard precautions, airborne precautions include patient placement in a negative pressure room, use of respiratory protection such as an N95 respirator, and limitation of patient transport.

Droplet Precautions

Droplets can be transmitted from coughing, sneezing, and talking, and during certain procedures such as suctioning and bronchoscopy. Transmission is via the host's conjunctivae, nasal mucosa, or mouth. Droplets do not remain suspended in the air and as such ventilation is not needed. Do not confuse droplet precautions with airborne transmission. In addition to standard precautions, droplet precautions include placement of the patient in a private room, use of a mask (especially when within 3 feet of the patient), and limited patient transport.

Contact Precautions

Contact is the most frequent mode of transmission of nosocomial infections and is divided into direct- and indirect-contact transmission.
  • *Direct-contact* transmission involves body-to-body contact that results in the physical transfer of microorganisms, such as bathing or turning a patient.
  • *Indirect-contact* transmission involves a susceptible host touching a contaminated object, such as instruments, needles, or dressings or hands that are not washed and gloves that are not changed between patients. Gloves should always be used in contact precautions. Gowns should be worn if there will be body-to-body contact or the patient has diarrhea, an ostomy, or excessive wound drainage. Before leaving the room, remove gloves and gown and thoroughly wash hands; be sure to avoid contact with any contaminated surfaces.

BIOLOGICAL AGENT DESCRIPTIONS

This chapter covers the following biological agents:
  • Anthrax (cutaneous, gastrointestinal, and inhalational)
  • Botulism
  • Brucellosis
  • Food safety threats
  • Glanders
  • Melioidosis
  • Plague

- Psittacosis
- Q fever
- Smallpox
- Staphylococcal enterotoxin B
- Tularemia
- Typhus, epidemic
- Viral encephalitides
- Viral hemorrhagic fevers
- Water safety threats

(For information on category C agents, see Chapter 4.)
For each agent, the following information is provided:

- Diagnosis synopsis
- Weaponization
- Transmission/isolation
- Incubation, duration, and mortality
- Patient assessment/recognition
- Clinical diagnostic tests
- Patient management
- Therapy
- Personal safety risk
- Precautions
- Family safety
- Vaccine
- Public health reporting

ANTHRAX

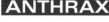

PERSONAL RISK   REPORTABLE DISEASE

BIOLOGICAL AGENT DESCRIPTION: ANTHRAX

OVERVIEW

Anthrax is a bacterial infection caused by *Bacillus anthracis*, an encapsulated, gram-positive, spore-forming bacterium. *B. anthracis* is present in both domestic and wild animals throughout the world and can be transmitted by their meat, wool, or hides. The spores are resistant to heat, UV light, microwave radiation, and many disinfectants. *B. anthracis* has been classified by the CDC as a category A bioterrorism agent because of its high lethality, hardiness, and ease of weaponization. In 2001 there were 22 cases of anthrax as a result of a bioterrorist attack. In 2002 the U.S. Department of Defense reintroduced the vaccination of military personnel and essential emergency civilians against anthrax.

There are three forms of anthrax:

1. Cutaneous
2. Gastrointestinal
3. Inhalational

Each is discussed separately on the following pages.

CUTANEOUS ANTHRAX

DIAGNOSIS SYNOPSIS

Although inhalational and gastrointestinal forms of anthrax exist, approximately 95% of all anthrax cases are cutaneous. Before 2001 there had not been a case of cutaneous anthrax reported in the United States since 1992. In the September 11, 2001 attacks, 11 of the 22 cases were cutaneous.

WEAPONIZATION

Cutaneous contact with aerosolized spores.

INCUBATION, ONSET, AND MORTALITY

- Incubation: 1 to 12 days
- Onset: 1 to 2 days
- Mortality: with treatment, <1%; without treatment, 20%

TRANSMISSION/ISOLATION

- Infection through cut or abrasion on the skin or handling infected animal products
- No person-to-person transmission
- Isolation not necessary

Biological Agents

PATIENT ASSESSMENT/RECOGNITION

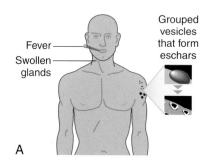

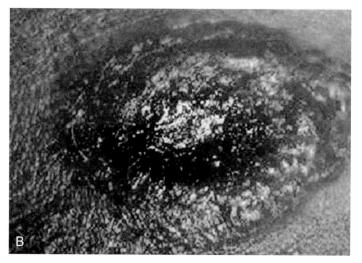

Cutaneous anthrax lesions evolve from pruritic papules to clusters of vesicles to ulcers within 1 to 2 days following exposure of abraded skin or wounds to the spores. The ulcers then develop into depressed black eschar over the next 2 to 5 days. The most common areas affected are the arms, face, and neck. Lymphangitis and painful lymphadenopathy are common.

With antibiotic treatment the death rate for cutaneous anthrax is approximately 1%. However, without treatment it may progress to a systemic form of anthrax with a death rate of approximately 20%. In these cases, the spores introduced into the body are eaten by macrophages and taken to regional lymph nodes, where they germinate into bacteria. Released into the lymph system, they enter the bloodstream, causing septicemia that results in a fatal toxemia.

CLINICAL DIAGNOSTIC TESTS

- Gram stain
- Blood culture
- Polymerase chain reaction (PCR)

PATIENT MANAGEMENT

- Notify your local department of health to inform them of a patient with *suspected* anthrax and to obtain any additional instructions *before* performing diagnostic tests.
- Initiate treatment based on a history of exposure or contact, not laboratory test results.
- Obtain specimens for culture; then notify your local laboratory regarding suspected anthrax and inform the laboratory that samples will be sent shortly.
- Do not use extended-spectrum cephalosporins or trimethoprim/sulfamethoxazole because anthrax may be resistant to these drugs.

THERAPY

See Table 6-3 for drug therapy.

PERSONAL SAFETY RISK

 Low risk to personal safety.

PRECAUTIONS

Standard precautions. Avoid direct contact with lesion(s) or lesion drainage.

FAMILY SAFETY/LEAVING WORK

 Low: Cutaneous anthrax is not contagious.

Biological Agents

TABLE 6-3	Therapy for Cutaneous Anthrax	
	ADULT	**CHILDREN**
Ciprofloxacin	500-mg oral tablet every 12 hr	20-30 mg/kg every 12 hr; do not exceed 1 g/day
Doxycycline	100-mg oral tablet every 12 hr	If >45 kg: same as adult If <45 kg: 2.5 mg/kg every 12 hr
Amoxicillin	500-mg oral pill every 8 hr	Depends on body weight

VACCINE
Vaccine is available.

GASTROINTESTINAL ANTHRAX

DIAGNOSIS SYNOPSIS
Gastrointestinal anthrax is rare; it is caused by consuming contaminated meat products and results in inflammation of the gastrointestinal (GI) tract.

For the purposes of biological warfare, GI anthrax would be placed in the food supply. Some countries have already experimented with this agent; both Japan and the former apartheid government of South Africa created anthrax-laced chocolates. The last reported case of GI anthrax in the United States was in 2000.

WEAPONIZATION
Contamination of food supply.

INCUBATION, ONSET, AND MORTALITY
- Incubation: 1 to 7 days
- Onset: within 7 days
- Mortality: 25% to 60%

TRANSMISSION/ISOLATION
- Consumption of infected/undercooked meat
- No person-to-person transmission
- Isolation not necessary

PATIENT ASSESSMENT/RECOGNITION

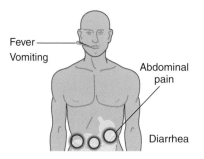

Symptoms of gastrointestinal anthrax include fever, anorexia, abdominal pain, ascites, bloody vomit, and diarrhea.

CLINICAL DIAGNOSTIC TESTS
- Gram stain
- Blood culture

PATIENT MANAGEMENT
- Notify your local department of health to inform them of the patient with *suspected* gastrointestinal anthrax and to obtain any additional instructions *before* performing diagnostic tests.
- Initiate treatment based on a history of exposure or contact, not laboratory test results.
- Obtain specimens for culture; then notify your local laboratory regarding suspected gastrointestinal anthrax and inform the laboratory that samples will be sent shortly.
- Antimicrobial therapy is critical during the early stages.
- Do not use extended-spectrum cephalosporins or trimethoprim/ sulfamethoxazole because anthrax may be resistant to these drugs.

THERAPY
See Table 6-4 for drug therapy.

PERSONAL SAFETY RISK

 Low risk to personal safety.

PRECAUTIONS
Standard precautions.

FAMILY SAFETY/LEAVING WORK

 Low: Gastrointestinal anthrax is not contagious.

TABLE 6-4	Therapy for Gastrointestinal Anthrax	
	ADULT	**CHILDREN**
Ciprofloxacin	500-mg oral tablet every 12 hr	20-30 mg/kg every 12 hr; do not exceed 1 g/day
Doxycycline	100-mg oral tablet every 12 hr	If >45 kg: same as adult If <45 kg: 2.5 mg/kg every 12 hr
Amoxicillin	500-mg oral pill every 8 hr	Depends on body weight

Biological Agents

VACCINE
Vaccine is available.

INHALATIONAL ANTHRAX

DIAGNOSIS SYNOPSIS

If anthrax were to be weaponized, the most likely method of dispersal would be by aerosol release, and although gastrointestinal and cutaneous forms of anthrax exist, inhalational anthrax would be the most likely to occur. In the 2001 terrorist attacks, 11 of the 22 cases were inhalational, resulting in 5 deaths. Before these attacks, the last reported case of inhalational anthrax was in 1976. A single case of inhalational anthrax may represent a bioterrorist threat and a public health emergency.

Extremely rare in normal circumstances, inhalational anthrax reaches a death rate of nearly 40% if treatment is not started in the prodromal phase.

WEAPONIZATION

Aerosol inhalation.

INCUBATION, ONSET, AND MORTALITY

- Incubation: 1 to 13 days
- Onset: 7 days
- Mortality: approximately 40%

TRANSMISSION/ISOLATION

- No person-to-person transmission
- Isolation not necessary

PATIENT ASSESSMENT/RECOGNITION

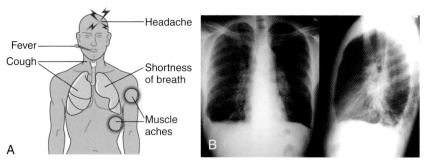

Look for nonspecific, flulike symptoms (e.g., low-grade fever, sweats, dry cough, headache, malaise, fatigue, dyspnea, and myalgias) in the first

24 to 48 hours with early chest radiography or computer tomography (CT) demonstrating a widened mediastinum and (often) pleural effusions. Infiltrates may also be present.

Initial symptoms are followed by a sudden onset of high fever and severe respiratory distress along with cyanosis, hypotension, shock, respiratory failure, and sudden death.

CLINICAL DIAGNOSTIC TESTS
- Chest x-ray (CXR)
- Gram stain
- Blood culture
- PCR

PATIENT MANAGEMENT
- Notify your local department of health to inform them of the patient with *suspected* inhalational anthrax and to obtain any additional instructions *before* doing diagnostic tests.
- Initiate treatment based on a history of exposure or contact, not laboratory test results.
- Obtain specimens for culture and notify your local laboratory regarding suspected anthrax and inform them that samples will be sent shortly.
- Early antibiotic therapy and cardio-respiratory support is critical; supportive therapy includes pleural effusions.
- Do not use extended-spectrum cephalosporins or trimethoprim/sulfamethoxazole because anthrax may be resistant to these drugs.

THERAPY
See Table 6-5 for drug therapy.

PERSONAL SAFETY RISK

 Low risk to personal safety.

PRECAUTIONS
Standard precautions.

FAMILY SAFETY/LEAVING WORK

 Low: Inhalational anthrax is not contagious.

Biological Agents

TABLE 6-5	Therapy for Inhalational Anthrax	
	ADULT	**CHILDREN**
Ciprofloxacin	500-mg oral tablet every 12 hr	20-30 mg/kg every 12 hr; do not exceed 1 g/day
Doxycycline	100-mg oral tablet every 12 hr	If >45 kg: same as adult If <45 kg: 2.5 mg/kg every 12 hr
Amoxicillin	500-mg oral pill every 8 hr	Depends on body weight

VACCINE
Vaccine is available.

BOTULISM

BIOLOGICAL AGENT DESCRIPTION: BOTULISM

DIAGNOSIS SYNOPSIS

Botulism is caused by a group of paralytic neurotoxins produced by the spore-forming, anaerobic, gram-positive bacillus *Clostridium botulinum*. Intoxication can occur naturally from contaminated foods or rarely as a result of wound or intestinal colonization in humans. There are seven types of botulinum toxins, A through G, although only A, B, E, and F have been implicated in the poisoning of humans. When used as a biological weapon, botulinum toxin is most likely to be dispersed as an aerosol for inhalation, although it could be added to the food or water supply. Botulinum toxins are, by weight, the most toxic agents known, with an LD50* of only 0.001 mcg/kg. Botulinum toxin irreversibly binds to the presynaptic cholinergic neuromuscular junction, blocking acetylcholine release and manifesting a symmetrical, progressive, descending flaccid paralysis after an 18- to 36-hour incubation period (occasionally up to several days). Multiple cranial nerve palsies are evident early in the course of the disease. Botulinum toxins are odorless and colorless in solution. Five minutes of heating the toxin above 85° C will inactivate the toxin. All materials suspected of containing toxin must be handled with caution. Before the shipment of any botulism-associated specimen, the designated laboratory must be notified and approved by the state health department.

*The lethal dose that results in the death of 50% of the subjects who are exposed to it.

WEAPONIZATION

- Aerosol inhalation
- Contamination of food and water supply

INCUBATION, ONSET, AND MORTALITY

- Incubation: 18 to 36 hours
- Onset: 6 hours to 2 weeks
- Mortality: overall, 5% to 10%; age older than 60 years, 30%

TRANSMISSION/ISOLATION

- No person-to-person transmission
- Isolation not necessary

PATIENT ASSESSMENT/RECOGNITION

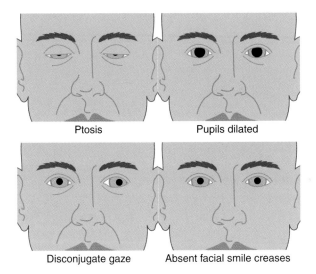

Ptosis   Pupils dilated

Disconjugate gaze   Absent facial smile creases

The hallmark symptoms of botulism are difficulty speaking, seeing, and/ or swallowing in combination with ptosis on exam. Also look for dilated (enlarged) and/or fixed pupils, diminished gag reflex, tongue weakness, and arm/leg weakness. The mouth may appear dry (xerostomia). The patient is afebrile.

CLINICAL DIAGNOSTIC TESTS

Sensitivity testing: brain scan, spinal fluid examination, nerve conduction test, and Tensilon test for myasthenia gravis (rules out similar diseases, such as Guillain-Barré syndrome).

Biological Agents

PATIENT MANAGEMENT

- Diagnosis primarily based on medical history and physical examination
- Supportive care and passive immunization with equine botulinum antitoxin (available from the CDC)

THERAPY

- Equine botulinum antitoxin
- Dose: dilute 10-ml vial, 1:10 in 0.9% saline solution; deliver IV slowly

PERSONAL SAFETY

 Low risk to personal safety.

PRECAUTIONS

Standard precautions.

FAMILY SAFETY/LEAVING WORK

 Low: Botulism is not contagious.

PROPHYLAXIS/VACCINE

Equine botulinum antitoxin.

BRUCELLOSIS

BIOLOGICAL AGENT DESCRIPTION: BRUCELLOSIS

DIAGNOSIS SYNOPSIS

Brucellosis is a systemic infection characterized by an undulant (intermittent) fever pattern. Typically a zoonotic infection of farm animals, the disease is produced in humans by infection with the gram-negative coccobacilli of the genus *Brucella*. Only four species of *Brucella* cause infection in humans: *B. melitensis* (goats and sheep), *B. ovis* (sheep and goats), *B. suis* (pigs), *B. abortus* (cattle), and rarely *B. canis* (dogs). *B. suis* and *B. melitensis* are the most common cause of brucellosis in humans. Weaponization of brucella is likely because of its ease of transmission by aerosol, and it is known to have been weaponized by several countries. During World War II the United States developed brucellosis as a biological weapon and dispersed it via bombs. Aerosolized brucella is highly infectious. In naturally occurring cases, human infection usually is caused by ingestion of contaminated dairy foods or infected animals (e.g., sheep, cattle, goats, or hogs) or through skin wounds.

WEAPONIZATION
Aerosol inhalation.

INCUBATION, ONSET, AND MORTALITY
- Incubation: 5 days to 6 months
- Onset: within 8 weeks
- Mortality: less than 2%

TRANSMISSION/ISOLATION
- Person-to-person transmission is rare.
- Isolation is not necessary.

CLINICAL DIAGNOSTIC TESTS
- PCR
- Antibody-based antigen detection systems
- Enzyme-linked immunosorbent assay (ELISA)
- Blood or bone marrow cultures

PATIENT ASSESSMENT/RECOGNITION

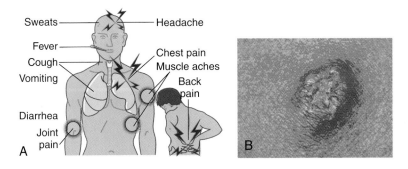

Brucellosis produces both an acute and a debilitating chronic illness. Typical acute systemic symptoms are nonspecific and flulike, and include undulant (intermittent) fevers, headache, chills, profuse sweating, malaise, myalgias, arthralgias, back pain, fatigue, anorexia, and irritability. GI symptoms are common and include nausea, vomiting, diarrhea, ileitis, colitis, and hepatitis. Other findings include bone pain caused by focal infection, pleuritic chest pain, and cough. Adenopathy, pharyngitis, and rash occur more commonly in children. Infection may progress to include the central nervous system (CNS) (meningitis) or the heart (endocarditis). Osteoarticular infections of the spine with paravertebral abscesses are common.

Medium and large joints are also commonly infected. Genitourinary involvement can lead to pyelonephritis, cystitis, and epididymo-orchitis. Infection with *Brucella* can lead to chronic painful symptoms lasting months. Death rates are less than 2%, and are often associated with endocarditis.

PATIENT MANAGEMENT
- Initiate therapy immediately.
- Administer doxycycline and rifampin in combination for 6 weeks to prevent reoccurring infection.
- Early treatment is critical; severity and duration of illness are dependent on timing of treatment.

THERAPY
See Table 6-6. Continue therapy for 6 weeks.

PERSONAL SAFETY RISK

 Low risk to personal safety.

PRECAUTIONS
Standard precautions.

TABLE 6-6	Therapy for Brucellosis	
	ADULTS	**CHILDREN**
Doxycycline	100 mg twice per day, oral	100 mg twice per day, oral
Rifampin	600 mg/day	15-20 mg/kg/day in one to two doses; maximum 600-900 mg/day

FAMILY SAFETY/LEAVING WORK

 Low: Brucellosis is not contagious.

VACCINE
None available.

FOOD SAFETY THREATS

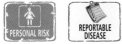

BIOLOGICAL AGENT DESCRIPTION: FOOD SAFETY THREATS

DIAGNOSIS SYNOPSIS
Foodborne diseases are caused by consuming contaminated food products. Many different disease-causing microbes as well as poisonous chemicals can contaminate foods. In fact, there are more than 250 known foodborne diseases, most of which are caused by a variety of bacteria, viruses, and parasites. Other diseases are poisonings, caused by harmful toxins or chemicals that have contaminated the food (e.g., poisonous mushrooms).

These different diseases have many different symptoms; however, since the microbe or toxin enters the body through the gastrointestinal tract, the first symptoms often include nausea, vomiting, abdominal cramps, and diarrhea.

Three foodborne diseases pose significant health threats:

1. *Escherichia coli* O157:H7
2. Salmonellosis
3. Shigellosis

WEAPONIZATION
Contamination of food supply.

INCUBATION, ONSET, AND MORTALITY
Each of these diseases has an incubation period of several days, and illness begins a few days following the exposure. Mortality is rare in all instances.

Biological
Agents

TRANSMISSION/ISOLATION

- Transmission occurs through consuming contaminated foods.
- Person-to-person transmission is rare.
- Isolation is not necessary.

PATIENT ASSESSMENT/RECOGNITION

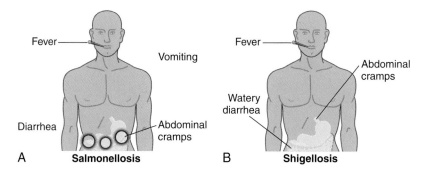

A   Salmonellosis   B   Shigellosis

Salmonellosis is caused by a group of gram-negative bacilli and results in mild to severe diarrheal disease. Serotypes *Salmonella typhimurium* and *S. enteritidis* are the most common in the United States, but *S. typhi* and *S. paratyphi* produce the most severe forms of the illness (typhoid and paratyphoid fevers, respectively).

The symptoms of nontyphoidal gastroenteritis include low-grade fever, chills, nausea, vomiting, diarrhea, and abdominal cramps.

The initial symptoms of typhoid and paratyphoid fevers include the acute or gradual onset of abdominal pain and tenderness, fever, chills, sweating, headache, anorexia, weakness, cough, sore throat, dizziness, and myalgias. It usually progresses to a severe illness with bacteremia and high fever that may last weeks. About 30% will develop a rash of erythematous papules on the trunk (rose spots) and 5% to 10% will suffer altered mental status. About 1% will develop bowel perforation.

Shigellosis (bacillary dysentery) is caused by the gram-negative bacteria *Shigella*, a member of the Enterobacteriaceae family. Two thirds of cases of shigellosis in the United States are caused by the *Shigella sonnei*, group D, bacterium. The remaining cases are caused by group B, *S. flexneri*. Infection with *S. flexneri* may result in Reiter syndrome, a chronic autoimmune condition producing arthralgia, eye problems, and dysuria.

About 1 to 3 days after exposure, the initial presentation will consist of fever, abdominal pain, cramping, and voluminous watery diarrhea. Dehydration may occur. Over 1 to 3 more days, the victim appears to improve with decreased fever and reduced diarrhea, but this is followed by toxemia (in Shiga's bacillus) with high fever, abdominal pain and tenderness, hyperactive bowel sounds, and rectal ulcerations. Without treatment, the illness can last up to 30 days (average of 7 days).

CLINICAL DIAGNOSTIC TESTS
- Gram stain
- Stool cultures
- Blood cultures

PATIENT MANAGEMENT
- Provide supportive therapy to hydrate patients.
- Patients usually recover in several days without additional treatment.

THERAPY
- Replace the lost fluids and electrolytes and keep up with fluid intake.
- If diarrhea is severe, administer an oral rehydration solution, such as CeraLyte, Pedialyte, or Oralyte, to replace the fluid losses and prevent dehydration.

PERSONAL SAFETY RISK

 Low risk to personal safety.

PRECAUTIONS
Standard precautions.

FAMILY SAFETY/LEAVING WORK

 Low: No threat to family.

VACCINE
None available.

Biological
Agents

GLANDERS

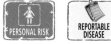

BIOLOGICAL AGENT DESCRIPTION: GLANDERS

DIAGNOSIS SYNOPSIS

Glanders is an infection caused by *Burkholderia mallei*, a gram-negative bacillus. It is typically an equine disease. Glanders has been classified by the CDC as a category B bioterrorism agent because of the moderate ease with which it can be disseminated. Infection can be localized to the skin (chronic glanders) or mucous membranes (acute localized glanders), or manifest in the pulmonary system (acute pulmonary) and it may begin as or progress to a septicemic form. The acute pulmonary form would be most likely following a bioterrorism attack. In acute localized glanders, the bacteria enter through breaks in the skin or mucosal surfaces of the eyes, nose, and mouth and cause conjunctivitis and/or bloody discharge of mucus and pus from the nose. Acute forms are almost always fatal without treatment. In chronic glanders, which has a delayed onset, cutaneous and intramuscular abscesses occur on the arms and legs. Splenic and liver abscesses may be seen as well as enlarged regional lymph nodes. On rare occasions, it progresses to meningitis.

WEAPONIZATION

Aerosol inhalation.

INCUBATION, ONSET, AND MORTALITY

- Incubation: 10 to 14 days
- Onset: abrupt
- Mortality: with treatment, 40%; without treatment, up to 95%

TRANSMISSION/ISOLATION

- Person-to-person transmission is possible, including sexual transmission.
- Isolate patients in a private room.

PATIENT ASSESSMENT/RECOGNITION

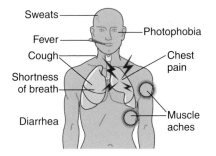

Whether acquired naturally (via inhalation or hematogenous spread) or as a result of a bioterrorist attack, pulmonary glanders has an incubation period of 10 to 14 days and presents with a sudden onset of flulike symptoms accompanied by fever, rigors, sweats, cough, chest pain, myalgias, lacrimation, diarrhea, photophobia, cervical adenopathy, splenomegaly, and a widespread papular/pustular rash similar to smallpox. It quickly progresses to pneumonia and/or pulmonary abscesses. Chest x-ray is positive for miliary nodules, infiltrates, and/or lung abscesses.

In acute localized glanders, the bacteria enter through breaks in the skin or mucosal surfaces of the eyes, nose, and mouth and cause conjunctivitis and/or bloody discharge of mucus and pus from the nose. Acute forms are almost always fatal without treatment.

In chronic glanders, which has a delayed onset, cutaneous and intramuscular abscesses occur on the arms and legs. Splenic and liver abscesses may be seen as well as enlarged regional lymph nodes. On rare occasions, it progresses to meningitis. Septicemic glanders is typically fatal within 7 to 10 days.

CLINICAL DIAGNOSTIC TESTS

- Gram stain
- Blood culture
- Sputum culture
- Urine culture
- Skin culture

PATIENT MANAGEMENT

- Mask suspected patients in the emergency department and during transport.
- Resistance to chloramphenicol has been reported.
- Limited information is available on treatment since human forms of glanders are rare.

Biological
Agents

TABLE 6-7	Therapy for Glanders
	TREATMENT
Adults	• Ceftazidime plus trimethoprim/sulfamethoxazole (TMP/SMX) for 2 weeks, IV • TMP/SMX oral therapy to complete at least a 6-month regimen
Children	• Ceftazidime 50 mg/kg IV every 8 hr

THERAPY
See Table 6-7 for drug therapy.

PERSONAL SAFETY RISK

 Low risk to personal safety.

PRECAUTIONS
Droplet precautions in addition to standard precautions.

FAMILY SAFETY/LEAVING WORK

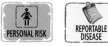 Low: Minimal risk since disease is not easily transmissible.

VACCINE
Prophylactic treatment: trimethoprim (TMP) 2 mg/kg and sulfamethoxazole (SMX) 10 mg/kg twice a day for at least 2 weeks.

MELIOIDOSIS

PERSONAL RISK   REPORTABLE DISEASE

BIOLOGICAL AGENT DESCRIPTION: MELIOIDOSIS

DIAGNOSIS SYNOPSIS
Melioidosis, or Whitmore's disease, is an infection caused by the gram-negative bacillus *Burkholderia pseudomallei*. The clinical presentation of melioidosis is similar to that for glanders (although it differs epidemiologically) and has been studied for potential weaponization in the past. Natural

occurrences of melioidosis are acquired through skin abrasions, inhalation, and other types of contact with contaminated water and soil. As an agent of bioterrorism, the most likely method of dispersal would be in an aerosolized form.

Melioidosis is usually nonfatal, except in the septicemic form. In a bioterrorism attack, death rates could be higher because of the higher initial bacterial exposure. There are four clinically distinct types of melioidosis: localized, pulmonary, septicemic, and chronic.

WEAPONIZATION
Aerosol inhalation.

INCUBATION, ONSET, AND MORTALITY
- Incubation: 2 days to 2 years
- Onset: abrupt or delayed
- Mortality: greater than 90% with septicemia

TRANSMISSION/ISOLATION
- Person-to-person transmission is possible, including sexual transmission.
- Isolate patients in a private room.

PATIENT ASSESSMENT/RECOGNITION

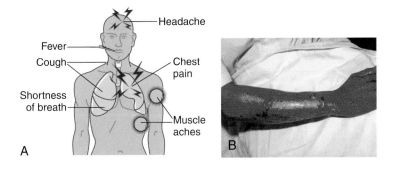

There are four clinically distinct types of melioidosis: localized, pulmonary, septicemic, and chronic.
- *Acute localized:* Acute localized melioidosis usually presents with a skin nodule or pustule. The skin lesions typically occur 1 to 5 days following an initial bacterial inoculation through a break in the skin from contaminated water or soil. Lymphadenitis and regional lymphadenopathy are common. Associated systemic symptoms may

include fever, chills, and myalgias. It may progress to septicemia, especially in immunocompromised patients or the chronically ill.

- *Pulmonary:* Pulmonary melioidosis has a clinical presentation that can vary from a mild bronchitis to a severe pneumonia. Symptoms occur 10 to 14 days after inhalation of aerosolized bacteria and include sudden onset of high fever, chills, productive or nonproductive cough, chest pain, headache, anorexia, and myalgia. This is the only form of melioidosis that presents with a cough. Skin abscesses may be seen, even months after infection, and it may produce late chronic lung abscesses that can be mistaken for cavitary tuberculosis (TB).

- *Septicemic:* Septicemic melioidosis usually results in septic shock and is most likely to occur in immunocompromised individuals and those with diabetes and renal insufficiency. Symptoms include headache, fever, chills, diarrhea, disseminated abscesses, myalgias, skin pustules, disorientation, and respiratory distress. Death rates are at least 90% and death may occur within 48 hours, even with therapy. Patients with diabetes, cirrhosis, lung disease, renal disease, or cystic fibrosis; the immunocompromised; and those who consume kava root are predisposed to septicemic infection.

- *Chronic suppurative:* Chronic suppurative melioidosis usually has a delayed onset and presents with abscesses in organs such as the skin, brain, liver, lungs, and spleen. It may also produce abscesses in the lymphatics, bones, and joints. It can produce a protracted wasting illness.

CLINICAL DIAGNOSTIC TESTS

- Gram stain
- Blood culture
- Sputum culture
- Urine culture
- Skin culture

PATIENT MANAGEMENT

- Early and rapid IV antibiotic therapy for severe disease is critical.
- Long-term prognosis is dependent on type of infection and course of therapy.

THERAPY

Treatment for 60 days:

Adults

- Ceftazidime 60 mg/kg IV or IM every 12 hours
- Plus: imipenem 500 mg IM or IV every 8-12 hours or amoxicillin-clavulanate 875 mg by mouth (PO) twice a day (bid)

Children
- Ceftazidime 60 mg/kg IV or IM every 12 hours
- Plus: imipenem 25 mg/kg IV every 6-8 hours (depending on age) or amoxicillin-clavulanate 30 mg/kg PO bid

PERSONAL SAFETY RISK

 Medium risk to personal safety.

PRECAUTIONS
Standard and contact precautions.

FAMILY SAFETY/LEAVING WORK

 Low: Change clothes to ensure that clothes are not contaminated.

VACCINE
None available.

PNEUMONIC PLAGUE

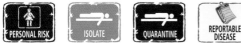

BIOLOGICAL AGENT DESCRIPTION: PNEUMONIC PLAGUE

DIAGNOSIS SYNOPSIS
Pneumonic plague is a severe bacterial lung infection caused by the gram-negative bacillus *Yersinia pestis. Yersinia pestis,* which is found in rodents (e.g., prairie dogs, squirrels, rats, etc.) and their fleas and sometimes in cats, can also cause other types of plague: bubonic and septicemic plague (bubonic plague associated with sepsis and delirium), either of which may progress to the pneumonic form. In a bioterrorist event, plague would most likely be released as an aerosol, resulting in the highly lethal and contagious pneumonic form of the illness. Whether pneumonic plague is acquired naturally or as a result of a bioterrorist attack, a severe fulminant illness develops that if not treated within 24 hours of onset can result in death.

Biological
Agents

WEAPONIZATION
Aerosol inhalation.

INCUBATION, ONSET, AND MORTALITY
- Incubation: 1 to 6 days
- Onset: abrupt
- Mortality: untreated, 50% to 90%; with treatment, 15%

TRANSMISSION/ISOLATION
- Pneumonic can be transmitted from person-to-person via droplets through direct, close contact.
- Isolate patients in a negative pressure room.
- Plague is a federally mandated quarantinable disease.

PATIENT ASSESSMENT/RECOGNITION

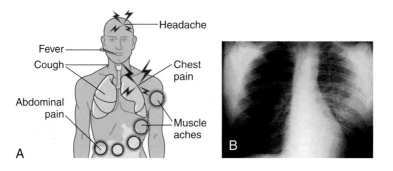

Pneumonic plague is a severe fulminant illness that develops with associated high fever, chills, headache, productive cough, chest pain, hemoptysis, extreme malaise, myalgias, tachypnea, tachycardia, and pneumonia. GI symptoms—nausea, vomiting, abdominal pain, and diarrhea—also are commonly seen.

If not treated within 24 hours of onset, pneumonic plague rapidly progresses to cyanosis, respiratory failure, septicemia, circulatory collapse, and death.

CLINICAL DIAGNOSTIC TESTS
- Blood culture
- Sputum culture
- Lymph node culture

PATIENT MANAGEMENT

- Begin treatment within 24 hours of initial symptoms.
- Identify and evaluate people closely associated with the patient and begin preventive antibiotic therapy if appropriate.
- Provide supportive care in the intensive care unit (ICU).

THERAPY

Streptomycin, gentamicin, the tetracyclines, or chloramphenicol for 7 days (Table 6-8).

TABLE 6-8	Therapy for Pneumonic Plague
PATIENT	**TREATMENT**
Adult	Streptomycin 1 g IM twice daily for 10 days (not in pregnant women)
	Or
	Gentamicin 5 mg/kg IM or IV once daily or 2 mg/kg loading dose followed by 1.7 mg/kg IM or IV tid for 10 days
	Or
	Doxycycline 100 mg IV twice daily or 200 mg IV once daily for 10 days (if gentamicin not available or oral antibiotics must be used)
	Or
	Ciprofloxacin 400 mg IV bid for 10 days (or other fluoroquinolones at appropriate dosing)
	Chloramphenicol (add for plague meningitis), 25 mg/kg IV 4 times daily for 10 days; concentrations should be maintained between 5 and 20 mcg/ml; concentrations greater than 25 mcg/ml can cause irreversible bone marrow suppression
Children	Streptomycin 15 mg/kg IM twice daily for 10 days (maximum daily dose 2 g)
	Or
	Gentamicin 2.5 mg/kg IM or IV tid for 10 days (adjust for renal function)
	Or
	Doxycycline: >45 kg, give adult dosage; <45 kg, 2.2 mg/kg IV twice daily for 10 days (maximum 200 mg/day)
	Or
	Ciprofloxacin 15 mg/kg IV bid for 10 days (maximum daily dose 1 g)
	Chloramphenicol (add for plague meningitis), 25 mg/kg IV 4 times daily for 10 days; concentrations should be maintained between 5 and 20 mcg/ml; concentrations greater than 25 mcg/ml can cause irreversible bone marrow suppression
	CONSULT SPECIALIST FOR DOSING

PERSONAL SAFETY RISK

 High risk to personal safety.

PRECAUTIONS

Airborne and droplet precautions in addition to standard precautions.

FAMILY SAFETY/LEAVING WORK

 Low: Change clothes to ensure that clothes are not contaminated.

VACCINE

Vaccine is no longer available in the United States.

PSITTACOSIS

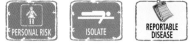

BIOLOGICAL AGENT DESCRIPTION: PSITTACOSIS

DIAGNOSIS SYNOPSIS

Psittacosis, also known as parrot disease, ornithosis, and chlamydiosis, is a rare zoonotic disease caused by the bacterium *Chlamydia psittaci* found in the dried secretions and droppings of wild and domestic birds and poultry. Natural infection occurs by inhalation of contaminated dust or aerosols, and as an agent of bioterrorism this would be the most likely method of dispersal.

Rarely, severe psittacosis can be fatal (less than 1% with proper antibiotic treatment). Death rates in a bioterrorism event may be higher because of a higher initial exposure.

C. psittaci is most commonly found in pet birds (e.g., parakeets, macaws, parrots, cockatiels), pigeons, ducks, and turkeys, which are often asymptomatic. Infected birds with symptoms present with diarrhea, shivering, sleepiness, anorexia, and breathing difficulties.

WEAPONIZATION

Aerosol inhalation.

Biological
Agents

INCUBATION AND MORTALITY
- Incubation: 5-15 days
- Mortality: with treatment, less than 1%; without treament, 15% to 20%

TRANSMISSION/ISOLATION
- Person-to-person transmission is rare.
- Transmission occurs through inhalation of aerosolized urine, dried droppings, and secretions from infected birds.
- Isolate patients in a private room.

PATIENT ASSESSMENT/RECOGNITION

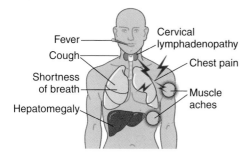

- Symptoms of psittacosis range from mild, nonspecific, and flulike to severe pneumonia with respiratory failure, and may include fever, chills, myalgias, headache, fatigue, chest pain, dry hacking cough, and shortness of breath. Crackles or rales may be present upon auscultation, and sputum may be blood tinged.
- Psittacosis may progress to include hepatic enlargement, splenic enlargement, cervical lymphadenopathy, urticaria, subungual hemorrhage, erythema nodosum, and erythema marginatum. Cardiac manifestations may include relative bradycardia, pericarditis, and myocarditis.
- A facial rash of pink macules (Horder's spots), similar to the rose spots of typhoid fever, may occur.
- Chest x-ray may show consolidation or patchy, miliary, or diffuse ground glass infiltrates.

CLINICAL DIAGNOSTIC TESTS
- Microimmunofluorescence
- Blood culture
- Sputum culture

- PCR
- Direct fluorescent antibody assay
- ELISA

PATIENT MANAGEMENT

- Mask suspected patients in the emergency department (ED) and during transport.
- Antibiotic treatment may prevent an antibody response, making diagnosis more difficult.
- Ask patients about recent exposure to birds.

THERAPY

Treatment for 10 to 21 days (Table 6-9).

PERSONAL SAFETY RISK

PERSONAL RISK Low risk to personal safety.

PRECAUTIONS

Droplet precautions in addition to standard precautions.

FAMILY SAFETY/LEAVING WORK

FAMILY RISK Low: Minimal risk since disease is not contagious.

VACCINE

None available.

TABLE 6-9	Therapy for Psittacosis
PATIENT	**TREATMENT**
Adults	• Doxycycline 100 mg PO or IV every 12 hr • Tetracycline 500 mg PO or IV qid
Children	• Doxycycline 2.5 mg/kg PO or IV every 12 hr • Tetracycline 6.25-12.5 mg/kg PO or IV qid

Q FEVER

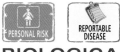

BIOLOGICAL AGENT DESCRIPTION: Q FEVER

DIAGNOSIS SYNOPSIS

Q fever is a zoonotic disease caused by the rickettsia-like organism *Coxiella burnetii*. Cattle, sheep, and goats are the primary reservoir, and transmission to humans typically occurs by direct contact with the body fluids of infected animals and with inhalation of *C. burnetii* in aerosolized body fluids and contaminated dust. Ingestion of contaminated milk or meat is a less common mode of transmission as are tick bites. *C. burnetii* is resistant to heat, drying, and common disinfectants, and very few organisms are required to cause illness. In a bioterrorism attack, the most likely method of dispersal would be as an aerosol release.

Chronic disease may develop and persist for over 6 months. The chronic form can occur up to 20 years after initial infection. The disease may progress to endocarditis or aseptic meningitis. Infection results in lifelong immunity and half of those infected remain asymptomatic.

WEAPONIZATION

Aerosol inhalation.

INCUBATION, ONSET, AND MORTALITY

- Incubation: 10 to 40 days
- Onset: abrupt
- Mortality: 1% to 2%

The incubation period of Q fever depends upon the number of organisms in the exposure, although 2 to 3 weeks is typical. It may be as short as 5 days following a massive exposure, as might be the case in a bioterrorism attack.

TRANSMISSION/ISOLATION

- Transmission through tick bites is rare.
- Person-to-person transmission has not been reported.
- Isolation is not necessary.

Biological
Agents

PATIENT ASSESSMENT/RECOGNITION

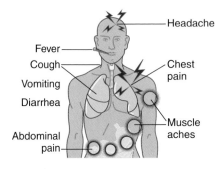

- Initial symptoms of Q fever include high fever (up to 104° F), chills, headache, malaise, myalgias, confusion, sore throat, sweats, nausea, vomiting, diarrhea, and abdominal pain. A pneumonia with nonproductive cough, chest pain, and rales may occur in 30% to 50% of cases after 4 to 5 days. Fever can persist for up to 2 weeks. Hepatitis may occur in some cases.
- Chronic disease may develop and persist for over 6 months. The chronic form can occur up to 20 years after initial infection. The disease may progress to endocarditis or aseptic meningitis.
- The prevalence of Q fever is unclear; half of those infected remain asymptomatic.

CLINICAL DIAGNOSTIC TESTS

- Indirect immunofluorescence assay (IFA)
- Immunohistochemical staining
- PCR
- CXR

PATIENT MANAGEMENT

- Treatment should be started immediately; it is most effective when started within the first 3 days of infection.
- Include supportive therapy in the form of IV fluids to manage weight loss.
- If disease relapses, restart therapy.

THERAPY

- Doxycycline
- Dose: 100 mg of doxycycline taken orally twice daily for 15 to 21 days

PERSONAL SAFETY RISK

 Low risk to personal safety.

PRECAUTIONS

Standard precautions.

FAMILY SAFETY/LEAVING WORK

 Low: Minimal risk since disease is not contagious.

VACCINE

Not available in the United States.

SMALLPOX

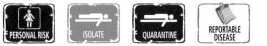

BIOLOGICAL AGENT DESCRIPTION: SMALLPOX

DIAGNOSIS SYNOPSIS

Smallpox is a contagious and often fatal infection caused by the variola virus. It presents in two clinical forms: variola major smallpox (historic death rate: 30%) and variola minor, which produces a milder smallpox-like illness (historic death rate: less than 1%). There are four clinical subtypes of smallpox: ordinary, modified, flat, and hemorrhagic; 90% of all smallpox cases were ordinary. Modified smallpox occurs in persons who have already been vaccinated against smallpox. Flat and hemorrhagic smallpox subtypes are very severe and rare. Smallpox, in all its forms, was declared eradicated in 1980 and there has not been a case since, but the virus still exists in some laboratories and may be in the hands of terrorists. Smallpox is classified as a category A bioterrorism agent because of its ease of dissemination, contagiousness, and high death rate. The most likely method of dispersal would be as an aerosol, but simply having an infected individual walk around infecting others is also a likely mode of dissemination. One case of smallpox most certainly represents a terrorist attack.

Biological Agents

Humans are the only known hosts of the variola virus. Smallpox is one of the most contagious diseases known, with only 5 to 10 virions sufficient to produce infection. Patients are most contagious from about 24 hours before the time the typical rash first appears until the scabs heal and fall off. During the incubation period it is not contagious. Although routine vaccination of children in the United States against smallpox was discontinued in 1972, beginning in 2002 military personnel and some clinicians, law enforcement personnel, public health officials, and other first responders have participated in a vaccination effort. Currently the vaccination is not available to the general public. The only people at risk for smallpox outside of a bioterrorist attack are those maintaining authorized stocks in laboratories at the CDC in Atlanta and in Moscow. Terrorist groups may be exposed if they are growing stocks of the virus for illicit purposes.

WEAPONIZATION
Aerosol inhalation.

INCUBATION, ONSET, AND MORTALITY
- Incubation: 3 to 17 days
- Onset: 2 to 4 days
- Mortality: variola major, 30%; variola minor, 1%

TRANSMISSION/ISOLATION
- It is easily spread person-to-person by respiratory droplets and/or contact with bodily fluids, lesions or scabs, and contaminated clothing or bedding.
- On rare occasions, in enclosed spaces, it has been transmitted by virus carried in the air.
- Patients are infectious from the onset of the rash until the last scab falls off.
- Isolate patients in a negative pressure room.
- Smallpox is a federally mandated quarantinable disease.

PATIENT ASSESSMENT/RECOGNITION

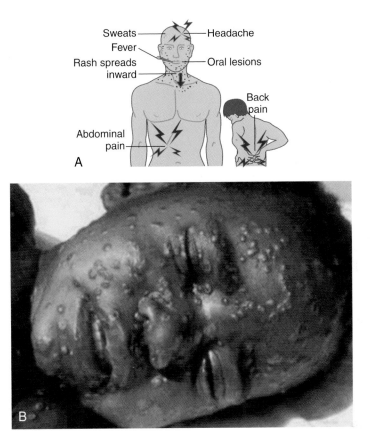

The initial symptoms of smallpox occur after a 3- to 17-day incubation period and include a prodrome of high fever, chills, headache, backache, malaise, and vomiting. Severe abdominal pain and delirium can also be present.

After 2 to 4 days a rash of macules and papules appears in the mouth and on the face and extremities and spreads inward to the rest of the body, including the palms and soles. The lesions of the rash evolve uniformly to vesicles and pustules, which usually umbilicate, crust over, scab, and fall off, leaving pitted scars.

After 2 weeks of infection, death can occur from a toxemia secondary to circulating immune complexes or from secondary infection. Encephalitis is a possible complication.

Hemorrhagic and flat forms are fulminant with death rates approaching 100% and do not display the typical umbilicated papules.

Biological Agents

- *Hemorrhagic smallpox:* In the hemorrhagic form of smallpox, petechiae and hemorrhage are associated with intense abdominal pain, headache, backache, and high fever.
- *Flat form:* In the flat form, constitutional symptoms are also severe, but the skin lesions are confluent, soft, red-orange papules that do not evolve into pustules and crusts.
- *Variola minor:* Variola minor has much less severe constitutional symptoms and fewer skin lesions.

CLINICAL DIAGNOSTIC TESTS

- Clinical presentation
- Electron microscopy
- PCR
- Antibody assays

PATIENT MANAGEMENT

- Quarantine patients immediately.
- Administer vaccine to prevent or lessen the disease; if rash is already present, vaccine will not protect individuals.
- Provide supportive therapy to manage symptoms.

THERAPY

- Provide supportive therapy with IV fluids, medicine to control fever or pain, and antibiotics for any secondary bacterial infections that may occur.
- Within 3 days of exposure: vaccine will prevent or greatly lessen the severity of the disease.
- Within 4 to 7 days of exposure: vaccine will offer some protection and/or decrease severity of disease.
- If rash is present: vaccine will not protect patient.

PERSONAL SAFETY RISK

 High risk to personal safety.

PRECAUTIONS

Airborne and contact precautions in addition to standard precautions.

FAMILY SAFETY/LEAVING WORK

 High: Remove and dispose of clothing and shoes as hazardous waste and decontaminate yourself before leaving work.

VACCINE

Vaccinia.

STAPHYLOCOCCAL ENTEROTOXIN B (SEB)

PERSONAL RISK   **REPORTABLE DISEASE**

BIOLOGICAL AGENT DESCRIPTION: STAPHYLOCOCCAL ENTEROTOXIN B (SEB)

DIAGNOSIS SYNOPSIS

Staphylococcal enterotoxin B (SEB) is a natural toxin produced by coagulase-positive *Staphylococcus aureus*. It produces one of the most common forms of food poisoning, and under natural conditions it is usually ingested when improperly stored food is eaten, producing a self-limited gastroenteritis. As a weapon, SEB would most likely be dispersed as an aerosol, producing an incapacitating but rarely lethal pulmonary and systemic syndrome. SEB was weaponized by the United States in the 1960s as an incapacitating agent. Via inhalation, the LD50* for SEB is approximately 0.02 mcg/kg. The CDC has assigned SEB as a category B bioterrorism agent (easy to produce and disseminate, moderate morbidity, low mortality).

In a bioterrorist attack, inhalation of higher concentrations may result in more severe symptoms such as dyspnea, chest pain, pulmonary edema, and/or acute respiratory distress syndrome (ARDS).

WEAPONIZATION

- Aerosol inhalation
- Contamination of food or water supply

INCUBATION, ONSET, AND MORTALITY

- Incubation: ingested, 4 to 10 hours; inhaled, 3 to 20 hours
- Onset: abrupt
- Mortality: rare

*The lethal dose that results in the death of 50% of the subjects who are exposed to it.

Biological Agents

TRANSMISSION/ISOLATION

- No person-to-person transmission
- Isolation not necessary

PATIENT ASSESSMENT/RECOGNITION

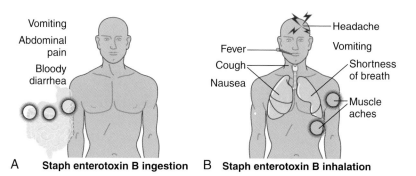

A   **Staph enterotoxin B ingestion**   B   **Staph enterotoxin B inhalation**

- *Ingestion:* Whether acquired naturally or as a result of a bioterrorist attack, if SEB is ingested the symptoms include nausea, vomiting, diarrhea, and abdominal pain/cramps.
- *Inhalation:* If SEB is inhaled, it presents with sudden onset of high fever (39.5° to 41° C), myalgias, chills, nonproductive cough, and headache. Conjunctivitis may also be noted. The fever may last 2 to 5 days and the cough may last for up to 4 weeks.
- Listen for moist rales on inhalation and exhalation. Chest x-ray is often normal, but may reveal Kerley's lines (interstitial edema), pulmonary edema, petechial hemorrhages, and atelectasis. A cluster of patients with unexplained pulmonary symptoms may be indicative of SEB.
- In a bioterrorist attack, inhalation of higher concentrations may result in more severe symptoms such as dyspnea, chest pain, pulmonary edema, and/or acute respiratory distress syndrome (ARDS).

CLINICAL DIAGNOSTIC TESTS

- Consider SEB in any cluster of patients with acute and unexplained respiratory illnesses.
- Differentiate from respiratory illnesses and exposures to toxic chemicals and other toxins, such as ricin.
- Perform serology on acute and convalescent serum.

PATIENT MANAGEMENT
- Provide supportive therapy of IV fluids, oxygen, and electrolytes.
- Intubation, mechanical ventilation, and measurement of positive end-expiratory pressure (PEEP) may be necessary.
- Patients usually recover from supportive therapy alone.

THERAPY
Supportive care with oxygen, IV fluids, and electrolytes.

PERSONAL SAFETY RISK

 Low risk to personal safety.

PRECAUTIONS
Standard precautions.

FAMILY SAFETY/LEAVING WORK

 Low: External decontamination is usually not required.

VACCINE
None available.

TYPHUS (EPIDEMIC)

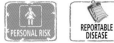

BIOLOGICAL AGENT DESCRIPTION: TYPHUS (EPIDEMIC)

DIAGNOSIS SYNOPSIS
Epidemic typhus (louse-borne typhus) is caused by infection with *Rickettsia prowazekii,* which is transmitted to humans by the body louse that lives within clothing and is found in conditions of poor hygiene. Wartime, famine or overcrowded conditions, and cold weather favor the proliferation of the louse vector. Infrequent clothing changes and bathing are a factor in louse proliferation. Mortality is variable, with increased mortality seen in the aged when there is a delay in antirickettsial therapy. If epidemic typhus were to be weaponized, the most likely method of dispersal

would be by aerosol release, but the release of infected lice is also a feasible alternative.

WEAPONIZATION

- Aerosol inhalation
- Release of infected lice
- Contamination of clothing

INCUBATION, ONSET, AND MORTALITY

- Incubation: 7 days
- Onset: abrupt
- Mortality: greater than 40%

TRANSMISSION/ISOLATION

- Is transmitted through the human body louse.
- Body lice are spread directly through contact with a person who has body lice, or indirectly through shared clothing, beds, bed linens, or towels.
- Isolation is not necessary.

PATIENT ASSESSMENT/RECOGNITION

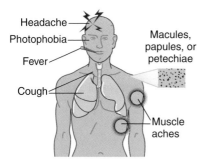

Whether acquired naturally or as a result of a bioterrorist attack, after a 7-day incubation period, the abrupt onset is heralded by an intense headache and fever. Chills, myalgias, and prostration are common, and a nonproductive cough may also be present. Fever rises to 39° C to 40° C (104° F) in an unremitting pattern. After 4 or 5 days of illness, a macular, papular, and/or petechial rash usually appears. Meningism is rarely reported. Central nervous system involvement may include confusion, delirium, and coma. Tinnitus and deafness have been reported. Renal insufficiency, pneumonia, and multiple organ failure may appear. Full recovery may take months.

TABLE 6-10	Therapy for Typhus
PATIENT	**TREATMENT**
Adults	• Doxycycline 100 mg PO every 12 hr • Tetracycline 500 mg PO qid • Chloramphenicol 12.5 mg/kg IV every 6 hr
Children	• Doxycycline 2.5 mg/kg PO every 12 hr • Tetracycline 6.25-12.5 mg/kg PO qid

CLINICAL DIAGNOSTIC TESTS
- PCR
- Weil-Felix test

PATIENT MANAGEMENT
If epidemic typhus is suspected, do not await laboratory confirmation to begin treatment.

THERAPY
Treatment for 2 to 3 additional days following defervescence (Table 6-10).

PERSONAL SAFETY RISK

 Low risk to personal safety.

PRECAUTIONS
Standard precautions.

FAMILY SAFETY/LEAVING WORK

 Low: Disease is not contagious.

VACCINE
None available.

Biological Agents

VIRAL ENCEPHALITIES

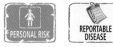

BIOLOGICAL AGENT DESCRIPTION: VIRAL ENCEPHALITIES

DIAGNOSIS SYNOPSIS

The viral encephalitides are mosquito-borne infections that include alphaviruses of the Togaviridae family and members of the Flaviviridae family.

- Togaviridae family: Venezuelan equine encephalitis (VEE), western equine encephalitis (WEE), eastern equine encephalitis (EEE)
- Flaviviridae family: St. Louis encephalitis, Japanese encephalitis, West Nile virus

Although the vast majority of natural infections occur as a result of a bite from an infected mosquito, these viruses are also infectious as aerosols and therefore could possibly be utilized as a bioterrorism weapon.

VEE would be the most likely candidate for weaponization as a result of its stability and ability to be highly infectious at a low dose. It also produces nearly 100% symptomatic infections. In addition, it has the potential to be altered genetically to produce a more virulent strain. Any outbreak of viral encephalitides in non-endemic areas or without preceding equine cases should be highly suspect for a bioterrorism attack.

WEAPONIZATION

Aerosol inhalation.

INCUBATION, ONSET, AND MORTALITY

- Incubation: 1 to 6 days
- Onset: abrupt or delayed
- Mortality: less than 1%

TRANSMISSION/ISOLATION

- The disease is transmitted via mosquitoes to humans and equines.
- Studies demonstrate that it can be transmitted via the aerosol route and therefore can be effectively weaponized.
- Direct person-to-person transmission via the aerosol route has been suggested but not proven.
- Isolation is not necessary.

PATIENT ASSESSMENT/RECOGNITION

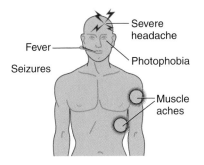

Whether acquired naturally or as a result of a bioterrorism event, symptoms of the viral encephalitides range from none to mild to severe and may include 24 to 72 hours of spiking fever, chills, fatigue, myalgias (especially in the low back), severe headache, and photophobia. Nausea, vomiting, sore throat, conjunctival redness, and diarrhea may quickly follow the initial onset of illness.

The disease may progress to CNS disturbances such as seizures, ataxia, paralysis, paresis, delirium, coma, and death. Severe CNS involvement is more common in children.

CLINICAL DIAGNOSTIC TESTS
- CBC
- ELISA
- Lumbar puncture

PATIENT MANAGEMENT
- Use standard precautions (gloves, hand washing, and splash precautions); a surgical or high efficiency particulate air (HEPA) filter (N-95 or better) mask may be helpful around coughing patients because of the uncertain risk of aerosol transmission.
- Because of possible transmission by the insect vector, control of mosquitoes is essential to prevent secondary cycles of infections.

THERAPY
- Provide supportive therapy with PO fluids, analgesics, and antiemetics.
- Severe cases may require anticonvulsants, IV fluids, and mechanical ventilation.

Biological
Agents

PERSONAL SAFETY RISK

 Low to medium, depending on presence of mosquito vectors and ambiguities in person-to-person transmission rate.

PRECAUTIONS

Standard precautions.

FAMILY SAFETY/LEAVING WORK

 Low: Minimal risk since viral encephalitides is not contagious.

VACCINE

- TC-83.
- Dose: single 0.5-ml subcutaneous dose
- C-84 (for those who already have TC-83 vaccine)
- Dose: 0.5-ml subcutaneous dose every 2 to 4 weeks, up to 3 doses or until an antibody response can be measured

VIRAL HEMORRHAGIC FEVERS

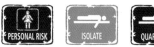

BIOLOGICAL AGENT DESCRIPTION: VIRAL HEMORRHAGIC FEVERS

DIAGNOSIS SYNOPSIS

Viral hemorrhagic fevers (VHFs) refer to a group of illnesses that are caused by four families of viruses that are classified as biosafety level four (BSL-4) pathogens. They cause a multisystem syndrome where the overall vascular system is damaged and the body is unable to repair itself. These symptoms are often accompanied by bleeding from the various orifices of the body. While some types of hemorrhagic fever viruses can cause relatively mild illnesses, many of these viruses cause severe, life-threatening disease.

Viruses causing VHFs are grouped in four families—arenaviruses, bunyaviruses, flaviviruses, and filoviruses:

Arenaviruses
- Argentine hemorrhagic fever (HF)
- Bolivian HF
- Sabia-associated HF
- Venezuelan HF
- Lassa fever
- Lymphocytic choriomeningitis

Bunyaviruses
- Crimean-Congo HF
- Hantavirus pulmonary syndrome
- Hemorrhagic fever with renal syndrome
- Rift Valley fever

Flaviviruses
- Kyasanur Forest disease
- Omsk HF
- Tick-borne encephalitis

Filoviruses
- Ebola HF
- Marburg HF

WEAPONIZATION

Aerosol inhalation.

INCUBATION, ONSET, AND MORTALITY

See Table 6-11 for incubation, onset, and mortality of viruses causing VHFs.

Biological Agents

TABLE 6-11	Incubation, Onset, and Mortality of Viruses Causing VHFs		
VIRUS	**INCUBATION**	**ONSET**	**MORTALITY**
Ebola	2-21 days	Abrupt	Up to 90%
Marburg	2-14 days	Abrupt	25%-90%
Lassa fever	3-16 days	1-3 weeks	15%-20% of symptomatic cases
Hantavirus	1-6 weeks	Abrupt	5%
Crimean-Congo	7-12 days	Abrupt	20%-50%
Rift Valley fever	2-6 days	Few days	1%
Tick-borne encephalitis	7 and 14 days	Few days	1%-2%

TRANSMISSION/ISOLATION

- Can occur by contact with urine, fecal matter, saliva, or other body excretions from infected rodents.
- Person-to-person transmission through close contact with infected people, the body fluids of infected individuals, or corpses is another mode of transmission.
- Isolate patients in negative pressure room.
- VHFs are federally mandated quarantinable diseases.

PATIENT ASSESSMENT/RECOGNITION

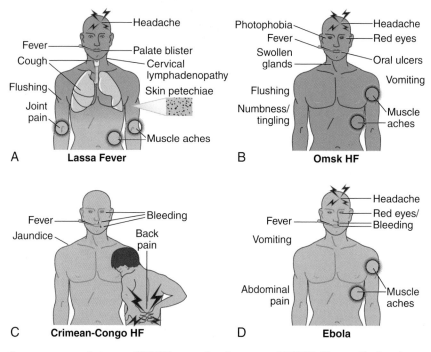

A   Lassa Fever

B   Omsk HF

C   Crimean-Congo HF

D   Ebola

Symptoms and signs of VHFs vary by the type of VHF. Typically, however, initial symptoms include fever, fatigue, dizziness, myalgias, loss of strength, and exhaustion.

Bleeding under the skin, in internal organs, or from the mouth, eyes, or ears may be seen in severe cases as well as shock, nervous system malfunction, coma, delirium, and seizures.

CLINICAL DIAGNOSTIC TESTS

- Electron microscopy
- CBC
- Virus culture

PATIENT MANAGEMENT
Supportive therapy through hydration, oxygen support, and electrolytes.

THERAPY
See Table 6-12 for drug therapy for VHFs.

TABLE 6-12	Therapy for VHFs by Type of HF
HF	**TREATMENT**
Argentine HF	Supportive FFP and platelets for hemorrhaging IV ribavirin may be helpful if begun before day 7 of illness, 30 mg/kg loading dose, then 15 mg/kg q6hr for 4 days, then 7.5 mg/kg q8hr for 6 days
Crimean-Congo HF	Supportive therapy with IV fluids and colloids as needed Management of coagulopathy with FFP and platelets Ribavirin IV 30 mg/kg loading dose, then 15 mg/kg q6hr for 4 days, then 7.5 mg/kg q8hr for 6 additional days may be helpful Interferon and convalescent human plasma may also be helpful, but have not been sufficiently tested
Ebola and Marburg	No specific therapy, though human convalescent plasma may be helpful Treatment is supportive only and management of coagulopathy with platelets and FFP has been somewhat successful
Hantavirus pulmonary syndrome	Supportive Management of airway ventilator
Kyasanur Forest disease	Supportive with IV fluids and whole blood Give FFP, platelets, and vitamin K to control hemorrhaging Avoid use of aspirin and other NSAIDs because of bleeding potential
Lassa fever	IV ribavirin 30 mg/kg loading dose, then 15 mg/kg q6hr for 4 days, then 7.5 mg/kg q8hr for 6 more days Treatment most effective if administered within 7 days of onset of symptoms Convalescent human serum effective if begun before day 9 of illness Supportive treatment
Omsk HF	Supportive Treat coagulopathy with FFP, platelets, and vitamin K
Rift Valley fever	Supportive Ribavirin may be helpful

FFP, Fresh frozen plasma; NSAID, nonsteroidal antiinflammatory drug.

Biological Agents

PERSONAL SAFETY RISK

 High risk to personal safety.

PRECAUTIONS

For Ebola, Marburg, Lassa fever, Hantavirus, and Crimean-Congo, use *all precautions.*

FAMILY SAFETY

 High: Remove and dispose of clothing and shoes as hazardous waste and decontaminate yourself before leaving work.

VACCINE

None available.

WATER SAFETY THREATS

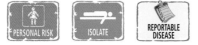

BIOLOGICAL AGENT DESCRIPTION: WATER SAFETY THREATS

DIAGNOSIS SYNOPSIS

Waterborne diseases are caused by drinking contaminated water or using contaminated water to cook food. There are several different agents that can contaminate water supplies. Just as is the case with foodborne illnesses, since the microbe or toxin enters the body through the gastrointestinal tract, the first symptoms often include nausea, vomiting, abdominal cramps, and diarrhea. Two of the most important waterborne diseases are cholera and cryptosporidium. Both diseases can last several weeks; however, illness from cholera can be more severe and requires immediate treatment.

WEAPONIZATION

Contamination of the water supply.

INCUBATION, ONSET, AND MORTALITY

Cholera
- Incubation: 4 hours to 5 days
- Onset: abrupt
- Mortality: high, if patient is not hydrated

Cryptosporidium
- Incubation: 5 to 6 days
- Onset: 2 to 10 days
- Mortality: rare

TRANSMISSION/ISOLATION

- Can occur by drinking water or using water for cooking that has been contaminated.
- Isolation is necessary for cases of cholera.
- Cholera is a federally mandated quarantinable disease.

PATIENT ASSESSMENT/RECOGNITION

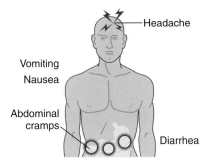

Headache

Vomiting
Nausea

Abdominal
cramps

Diarrhea

Cholera: Symptoms may be mild or severe with asymptomatic cases occurring frequently. Symptoms include abdominal cramping, severe watery gray-brown (rice water) diarrhea, vomiting, malaise, and headache. Fever occurs infrequently. Fluid loss may approach 1 L per hour and dehydration secondary to the diarrhea can result in circulatory collapse and shock in some cases. Without treatment, the symptoms last from 1 to 7 days, with death rates as high as 50%.

CLINICAL DIAGNOSTIC TESTS

- Stool culture
- Dark-field or phase contrast microscopy

Biological
Agents

PATIENT MANAGEMENT
- Hydrate patients immediately.
- In the case of cholera, the rapid loss of body fluids leads to dehydration, shock, and death if not treated.

THERAPY
- Oral hydration and/or IV hydration with fluid and balanced glucose-electrolyte solution. Glucose-electrolyte solution should contain 1 L of water plus 20 g of glucose, 3.5 g of NaCl, 2.5 g of sodium bicarbonate, and 1.5 g of KCl.
- Ciprofloxacin 10-15 mg/kg (up to 1 g) PO as a single dose or 500 mg PO bid for 3 days
- Doxycycline 300 mg PO as a singe dose or 100 mg PO bid for 3 days
- If resistant to tetracycline:
  - TMP-SMX
  - Erythromycin
  - Chloramphenicol

PERSONAL SAFETY RISK

Low risk to personal safety.

PRECAUTIONS
Standard precautions. **NOTE:** In an outbreak of cholera, appropriate disposal of feces, frequent hand washing, and efforts to maintain clean food and water supplies are imperative. *Vibrio cholerae* shedding in feces continues for 1 to 2 weeks after infection.

FAMILY SAFETY/LEAVING WORK

Low risk to family safety.

VACCINE
None available.

Radiological and Nuclear Disasters

CRITICAL INFO

- Notify your state radiation control program director.
- Consult with your institution's radiation safety officer or radiation physicist to determine type of radiation exposure.
- Triage allocation of scarce resources is imperative.
- Contact one or more of the following agencies for more information:
  - Radiation Emergency Assistance Center/Training Site (REAC/TS) at 1-865-576-3131 (M-F, 8 AM to 4:30 PM EST) or 1-865-576-1005 (after hours)
  - The Armed Forces Radiobiology Research Institute, Medical Radiobiology Team, at 1-301-295-0530
  - Centers for Disease Control and Prevention at 1-800-CDC-INFO

OVERVIEW

Radiation is a form of energy that is present all around us. It is found naturally in the sun, soil, and rocks, as well as in manmade objects such as television sets, microwave ovens, and medical and dental x-rays. Radiation cannot be detected by sight, smell, or any other sense. Radioactive materials are dangerous because of the harmful effect of certain types of radiation on the cells of the body. Therefore a person's risk increases the longer the person is exposed to radiation. It is important to note, however, that even though a person may be exposed, that person may not be contaminated. Similarly, a person may be contaminated with radioactive materials but may not be radioactive.

A radiological disaster may be the result of an accident occurring at a nuclear power plant, as in the case of the Chernobyl disaster in 1987, or the detonation of a nuclear weapon, as in the case of Hiroshima and Nagasaki in 1945. It may also be the result of a terrorist attack.

MEASURING RADIATION EXPOSURE

When a person is exposed to radiation, energy is deposited on the person. The amount of energy deposited per unit of weight of human tissue is called the absorbed dose. Absorbed dose is measured using the conventional radiation absorbed dose (rad) or the Gray (Gy). One Gy is equal to 100 rad.

Radiological and Nuclear Disasters

THREE WAYS TO MINIMIZE RADIATION EXPOSURE

- *Distance.* The greater the distance between you and the source of the radiation, the less radiation you will receive.
- *Shielding.* The greater the heaviness and denseness of the materials between you and the source of the radiation, the less radiation you will receive. The walls in your home may be sufficient shielding to protect you in the event of an emergency.
- *Time.* Limiting the time spent near the source of radiation reduces the amount of radiation you will receive since most radioactivity loses its strength fairly quickly.

ESTABLISHING A TRIAGE AREA

- Maintain a safe distance from the explosion.
- The anticipated number of casualties should be considered when choosing a triage area.
- A buffer zone should separate a contaminated area from a clean area.
- Be alert for fires, exposed high-voltage wires, sharp or falling objects, tripping hazards, or any hazardous chemicals that may cause physical harm.
- Place radiation measuring instruments in plastic bags to prevent their contamination and use them to map the areas leading up to the highest dose rates.
- Wash vehicles before leaving the scene.
- Before leaving the scene, remove and discard your clothing and rinse your full body with lukewarm water to remove any contamination not already removed with the outer clothing, and then survey your body with a radiation meter.

PROTECTING YOURSELF ON-SCENE

- Wear a mask equipped with a high efficiency particulate air (HEPA) filter (if you have no mask, a surgical mask, wet handkerchief, or cloth will work).
- Wear loose-fitting clothes covering as much of your body as possible to prevent radioactive dust from coming into direct contact with your skin, especially open wounds or abrasions.
- Do not eat, drink, or smoke while exposed to potentially radioactive dust or smoke.
- Survey your hands and clothing with a radiation meter at regular intervals.

Radiological and
Nuclear Disasters

- Beware of heat strain since this might cause carelessness and inefficiency.
- Radioactive objects should be handled with forceps and placed in lead containers.
- Keeping adequate records of contact information for all exposed workers is necessary in order to give them proper medical examinations later.
- Pregnant staff should be reassigned to other areas.

PATIENT MANAGEMENT/ DECONTAMINATION PRINCIPLES

- Treat life-threatening injuries (nonradiation) first before assisting patients with radiation contamination.
- All patients should be surveyed at regular intervals with a radiation meter, and the location and level of exposure should be documented.
- Document timing of any prodromal signs and symptoms (e.g., nausea, vomiting).
- Draw an initial complete blood count and repeat every 4 to 6 hours to evaluate lymphocyte depletion.
- Cut and roll clothing away from the face, bag according to hazardous waste guidelines, and label with patient information.
- Wounds should be irrigated with saline or water and covered with water-proof dressing.
- Any eye, nose, ear, or mouth contamination should be flushed.
- Intact skin should be washed with soap and water, starting outside the contaminated area and moving inward.
- Washing should be repeated until radiation level is no more than twice the background level or if the level remains unchanged.
- In mass casualty events, establish separate shower areas for ambulatory and nonambulatory patients.

HEALTH EFFECTS OF RADIOLOGICAL AND NUCLEAR INCIDENTS

OVERVIEW

The detonation of a nuclear or radiological device can have devastating health consequences on those exposed to the event. The severity of the injury or condition will be dependent on several factors: distance to the exposure, length of the exposure, and material composition of the device. This chapter will examine the health effects caused by acute radiation syndrome, cutaneous radiation injury, radiological dispersal device ("dirty bomb") injuries, and nuclear blast injuries.

MEDICAL COUNTERMEASURES

Three countermeasures exist to treat the health effects of a nuclear or radiological incident depending on the chemical composition of the exposure:
- Potassium iodide
- Diethylenetriaminepentaacetate
- Prussian blue

POTASSIUM IODIDE (KI)

KI is a salt of iodine. It can be used in the event of a nuclear incident as a "blocking agent" to prevent the human thyroid gland from absorbing radioactive iodine. If a nuclear incident occurs, officials will need to determine whether or not radioactive substances were present in the explosive device before recommending that people take KI. Some important considerations for using KI are as follows:
- KI is only effective if radioactive iodine is present.
- KI must be used immediately after the exposure occurred.
- Generally, KI should only be administered once. Exception: If a person expects to be exposed to radioactive iodine for more than 24 hours, another dose should be taken every 24 hours.
- KI may still have some protective effect even after 3 to 4 hours after exposure; however, the protective effect will not be as great and will continue to decrease as time passes (Table 7-1).
- KI will only protect the thyroid gland from radioactive iodine; it will not protect other parts of the body.
- For more specific information regarding KI administration, please consult the individual health effects that follow.

People should not take KI if any of the following conditions exist:
- History of thyroid disease
- Presence of iodine allergy
- Presence of certain skin disorders such as dermatitis herpetiformis or urticaria vasculitis

TABLE 7-1	KI Effectiveness Timeline	
HIGHLY PROTECTIVE	**EFFECTIVENESS DECEASES**	**<7% EFFECTIVE**
0-4 hours	5-24 hours	>24 hours

DIETHYLENETRIAMINEPENTAACETATE (DTPA)

DTPA is a calcium or zinc salt that is used to treat internal contamination by plutonium, americium, and curium. It binds to the radioactive material and accelerates the release of these materials in the urine. It is most effective when given within the first 24 hours after internal contamination. DTPA may still be administered effectively within several days or weeks following an exposure.

PRUSSIAN BLUE (RADIOGARDASE)

Prussian blue is used to treat people who have been internally contaminated with radioactive cesium and nonradioactive thallium. Prussian blue acts by containing the radioactive materials in the intestines and prevents them from being absorbed by the body. It can be administered at any point after it is determined that a person is internally contaminated.

ACUTE RADIATION SYNDROME

OVERVIEW

Acute radiation syndrome (ARS) is an acute illness caused by irradiation of the entire body, or most of the body, by a high dose of penetrating radiation in a very short time. The major cause of this syndrome is depletion of immature parenchymal stem cells in specific tissues. Examples of people who suffered from ARS are the survivors of the Hiroshima and Nagasaki atomic bombs and the firefighters that first responded after the Chernobyl nuclear power plant event in 1986. ARS is further divided into three classes (bone marrow, gastrointestinal [GI], and cardiovascular [CV]/central nervous system [CNS]) depending upon the radiation dose, which is measured in Gy (or rad) (Table 7-2).

TABLE 7-2	Estimation of External Radiation Dose Related to Onset of Vomiting*	
VOMITING POST INCIDENT	**ESTIMATED DOSE**	**DEGREE OF ARS**
Less than 10 minutes	>8 Gy	Lethal
10-30 minutes	6-8 Gy	Very severe
Less than 1 hour	4-6 Gy	Severe
1-2 hours	2-4 Gy	Moderate
More than 2 hours	<2 Gy	Mild

From http://www.orau.gov/reacts.
*For acute external exposures only. Gray (Gy) is the SI unit of measurement for radiation-absorbed dose.

EXPOSURES
- Atomic bomb
- Nuclear power plant disaster
- Unintentional exposures to sterilization irradiators

Bone Marrow Syndrome (Dose: 0.7-10 Gy)
Full recovery is expected in most cases.

Death may occur in some individuals at 1.2 Gy (120 rad) (Table 7-3).

The LD50/60 (lethal dose that results in the death of 50% to 60% of the subjects who are exposed to it) is about 2.5 to 5 Gy (250 to 500 rad).

Gastrointestinal Syndrome (Dose: >10 Gy)
Survival is extremely unlikely; death occurs within 2 weeks (Table 7-4).

Death is due to infection, dehydration, and electrolyte imbalance.

Cardiovascular/Central Nervous System
No recovery is expected; death occurs within 3 days (Table 7-5).

TABLE 7-3	Bone Marrow Syndrome	
PRODROMAL STAGE	**LATENT STAGE**	**MANIFEST ILLNESS STAGE**
Minutes to days	1-6 weeks	Few weeks to 2 years
Anorexia	Patient may appear	Anorexia
Nausea	and feel well	Fever
Vomiting		Malaise

TABLE 7-4	Gastrointestinal Syndrome	
PRODROMAL STAGE	**LATENT STAGE**	**MANIFEST ILLNESS STAGE**
2 days	<1 week	<1 week
Anorexia	Patient may appear	Anorexia
Severe nausea	and feel well	Fever
Vomiting		Malaise
Cramps		Severe diarrhea
Diarrhea		Dehydration
		Electrolyte imbalance

Radiological and Nuclear Disasters

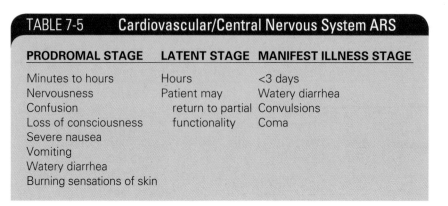

TABLE 7-5	Cardiovascular/Central Nervous System ARS	
PRODROMAL STAGE	**LATENT STAGE**	**MANIFEST ILLNESS STAGE**
Minutes to hours	Hours	<3 days
Nervousness	Patient may	Watery diarrhea
Confusion	return to partial	Convulsions
Loss of consciousness	functionality	Coma
Severe nausea		
Vomiting		
Watery diarrhea		
Burning sensations of skin		

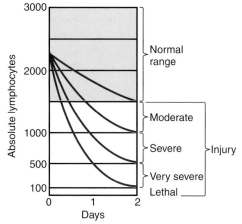

Figure 7-1. Andrews lymphocyte nomogram. (From Andrews GA, Auxier JA, Lushbaugh CC: The importance of dosimetry to the medical management of persons exposed to high levels of radiation. In *Personal dosimetry for radiation accidents,* Vienna, 1965, International Atomic Energy Agency.)

THERAPY

- Based on type of ARS, treat symptomatically, focusing on prevention of infection.
- Draw complete blood count (CBC) every 2 to 3 hours during the first 8 hours after exposure and every 4 to 6 hours for the next 48 hours (Figure 7-1).
- Closely monitor the lymphocyte count.

PERSONAL SAFETY RISK

  Low, since ARS is not contagious.

PRECAUTIONS
Standard precautions.

FAMILY SAFETY/LEAVING WORK

 Low: Change clothing, including shoes, and shower to remove any radioactive dust before going home.

CUTANEOUS RADIATION INJURY

OVERVIEW
Cutaneous radiation injury (CRI) refers to an injury to the skin and underlying tissues from acute exposure to a large external dose of radiation. Acute radiation syndrome will usually be accompanied by some skin damage; however, CRI can occur without symptoms of ARS. This is especially true with acute exposures to beta radiation or low-energy x-rays, because beta radiation and low-energy x-rays are less penetrating and less likely to damage internal organs than gamma radiation. CRI can occur with radiation doses as low as 2 Gray (Gy) or 200 rad, and the severity of CRI symptoms will increase with increasing doses.

EXPOSURES
- Unsecured radiation sources from food irradiators
- Radiotherapy equipment
- Well depth gauges
- Overexposed to x-radiation from fluoroscopy units

Grade I (Dose: >2 Gy)
Complete healing expected 28 to 40 days, 3 to 6 months post exposure (Table 7-6)
Slight atrophy of the skin possible
Possible skin cancer in decades following exposure

Grade II (Dose: >15 Gy)
Healing and recovery dependent on the magnitude of the injury and the possibility of more cycles of erythema
Possible skin atrophy or ulcer recurrence
Possible telangiectasia (up to 10 years post exposure) (Table 7-7)
Possible skin cancer in decades following exposure

TABLE 7-6	Grade I Cutaneous Radiation Injury		
PRODROMAL STAGE	**LATENT STAGE**	**MANIFEST ILLNESS STAGE**	**THIRD WAVE OF ERYTHEMA**
Minutes to days	2-5 weeks	20-30 days	Few weeks to months
Not apparent	Not apparent	Redness of skin Slight edema Possible increase in pigmentation Dry desquamation	Not apparent

TABLE 7-7	Grade II Cutaneous Radiation Injury		
PRODROMAL STAGE	**LATENT STAGE**	**MANIFEST ILLNESS STAGE**	**THIRD WAVE OF ERYTHEMA**
1-2 days Immediate sensation of heat	<2 weeks Not apparent	8 weeks Redness of skin Blisters Sense of heat Slight edema Possible increased pigmentation Erosions Ulceration Severe pain	Months to years Injury of blood vessels Edema New ulcers Increasing pain Possible necrosis

Grade III (Dose: >40 Gy)

Recovery can involve ulcers that are extremely difficult to treat and can require months to years to heal fully.

Possible skin atrophy, depigmentation, constant ulcer recurrance, or deformity

Possible occlusion of small vessels with subsequent disturbances in blood supply, destruction of the lymphatic network, regional lymphostasis, and increasing fibrosis and sclerosis of the connective tissue

Possible telangiectasia

Possible skin cancer in decades following exposure

Grade IV (Dose: >550 Gy)

Recovery possible following amputation of severely affected areas and possible skin grafts

TABLE 7-8	Grade IV Cutaneous Radiation Injury		
PRODROMAL STAGE	**LATENT STAGE**	**MANIFEST ILLNESS STAGE**	**THIRD WAVE OF ERYTHEMA**
Minutes to hours	<4 days	Several weeks	N/A
Immediate pain or tingling, accompanied by swelling	Not apparent	Early ischemia (tissue turns white, then dark blue or black with substantial pain) Necrotic tissue within 2 weeks post exposure Substantial pain Blisters	Does not occur because of necrosis of skin in affected area

Plastic surgery may be required over several years
Possible skin cancer in decades following exposure (Table 7-8)

THERAPY

- Treat localized injuries symptomatically, focusing on pain and infection control.
- Within 48 hours of injury, wounds should be closed, burns covered, fractures reduced, surgical stabilization performed, and definitive treatment given.
- After 48 hours, surgical intervention should be delayed until hematopoietic recovery has occurred.

PERSONAL SAFETY RISK

 Low, since CRI is not contagious.

PRECAUTIONS

Standard precautions.

FAMILY SAFETY/LEAVING WORK

 Low: Change clothing, including shoes, and shower to remove any radioactive dust before going home.

Radiological and Nuclear Disasters

RADIOLOGICAL DISPERSAL DEVICE ("DIRTY BOMB") INJURIES

OVERVIEW

A "dirty bomb" is a mix of explosives, such as dynamite, with radioactive powder or pellets. When the dynamite or other explosives are triggered, the blast carries radioactive material into the surrounding area. A dirty bomb is completely different from an atomic bomb because the dirty bomb uses dynamite or other explosives to scatter radioactive dust or smoke in order to radioactively contaminate its victims. An atomic bomb, on the other hand, involves the splitting of atoms, which, in turn, releases a huge amount of energy and produces a mushroom cloud.

PATIENT ASSESSMENT/RECOGNITION

Low levels of radiation exposure: no symptoms
Higher levels of radiation exposure:
    GI: nausea, vomiting, diarrhea
    Skin: swelling and redness

DIAGNOSTIC TESTS

- Survey patients with a Geiger-Müller detector to determine exposure dosage.
- Survey patients with an alpha meter if a life-threatening emergency is not identified.

PATIENT MANAGEMENT

- Tell patients to cover nose and mouth with cloth to prevent inhaling dust.
- Tell patients to remove clothing and place in plastic bag.
- Allow patients to take a shower with soap and water; make sure they wash their hair.
- Clean and cover any open wounds.

THERAPY

- Antinausea drugs and painkillers can relieve some symptoms.
- Antibiotics can fight secondary infections.
- Blood transfusions may be needed.

PERSONAL SAFETY

 May be high, depending on the fallout.

PRECAUTIONS
Standard precautions.

FAMILY SAFETY/LEAVING WORK

 Low: Change clothing, including shoes, and shower to remove any radioactive dust before going home.

PROPHYLAXIS
Investigators should first determine whether radioactive iodine was used in the explosive device before administering KI. A "dirty bomb" generally will not contain radioactive iodine, so KI pills are of no use for a "dirty bomb."

NUCLEAR BLAST INJURIES

OVERVIEW
A nuclear blast is an explosion of a nuclear bomb, which involves the joining or splitting of atoms. This process results in the production of an intense wave of heat, light, air pressure, and radiation. Upon detonation of a nuclear device, a large fireball is created, vaporizing everything inside it. A mushroom cloud forms immediately afterwards.

The vaporized material in the mushroom cloud then mixes with the radioactive material from the nuclear device to form particles, which later fall back to the earth. This is what is known as fallout. Fallout can be carried long distances on wind currents, and since it is radioactive it can contaminate anything on which it lands, including food and water supplies.

The bombs dropped on Hiroshima and Nagasaki, Japan, at the end of World War II are examples of nuclear blasts.

EXPOSURES
- Atomic bomb
- Nuclear power plant disaster

PATIENT ASSESSMENT/RECOGNITION
- Skin: moderate to severe skin burns
- Eyes: eye damage ranging from temporary blindness to severe burns on the retina
- GI: radiation sickness (ARS)

DIAGNOSTIC TESTS

- CBC should be taken within 8 to 12 hours of the exposure to assess lymphocyte depletion and exposure dosage.
- Use chromosome aberration cytogenetic bioassay to confirm exposure dosage.

PATIENT MANAGEMENT AND THERAPY

- Secure airway, breathing, and circulation (ABC) and physiological monitoring (blood pressure, blood gases, electrolyte and urine output) as appropriate.
- Administer supportive care in a clean environment.
- Treat major trauma, burns, and respiratory injury if evident.

PERSONAL SAFETY

 May be high, depending on the fallout.

PRECAUTIONS

Standard precautions.

FAMILY SAFETY/LEAVING WORK

 Low: Change clothing, including shoes, and shower to remove any radioactive dust before going home.

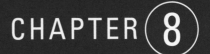

Explosives/Mass Casualty Events

CRITICAL INFO

- Maximize the number of lives saved.
- Ration supplies in a way to maximize the number saved.
- Expect reverse triage—less severely injured patients will arrive first.
- Ration supplies accordingly to ensure that most severely injured patients receive treatment.
- Wounds can be grossly contaminated; consider delayed primary closure and assess tetanus status; ensure close follow-up of wounds, head injuries, and eye-, ear-, and stress-related complaints.
- Communications and instructions may need to be written because of tinnitus and sudden temporary or permanent hearing loss.

OVERVIEW

There are multiple definitions of mass casualty events (MCEs), with numbers ranging from 100 to 1000. It should be considered an MCE anytime there is a sudden influx of injured or ill patients into the emergency department (ED) that overwhelms the hospital's resources. MCEs disrupt communication systems, interrupt transportation of both patients and supplies, and strain the financial and personnel abilities of agencies trying to handle the aftermath of the disaster. MCEs can also result in negative health effects caused directly by the incident, such as injuries or disabilities, as well as indirectly, such as in the case of substance abuse or psychological trauma.

NURSES' ROLE

- Rapid assessment of the situation and of nursing care needs
- Provision of disaster triage and initiation of life-saving measures first
- The ability to maximize the number of lives saved
- Ability to ration supplies in a way to maximize the number saved
- Selected use of essential nursing interventions and the elimination of nonessential nursing activities
- Adaptation of necessary nursing skills to disaster and other emergency situations
- Evaluation of the environment and the mitigation or removal of any health hazards
- Prevention of further injury or illness

- Leadership in coordinating patient triage, care, and transport during times of crisis
- The teaching, supervision, and utilization of auxiliary medical personnel and volunteers
- Adaptation to shortages in providers; ability to assume multiple roles
- Provision of understanding, compassion, and emotional support to all victims and their families
- Provision of documentation on patients to the best of ability

EXPLOSIONS AND BLAST INJURIES

Explosions can produce unique patterns of injury seldom seen outside combat. When they do occur, they have the potential to inflict multisystem life-threatening injuries on many persons simultaneously. The injury patterns following such events are a product of the composition and amount of the materials involved, the surrounding environment, the delivery method (e.g., bomb), the distance between the victim and the blast, and any intervening protective barriers or environmental hazards.

CLASSIFICATION OF EXPLOSIVES

See Table 8-1 for descriptions and examples of types of explosives.

MECHANISMS OF BLAST INJURIES

See Table 8-2 for categories of blast injuries, including body part affected and type of injury.

TABLE 8-1	Types of Explosives	
EXPLOSIVE TYPE	**DESCRIPTION**	**EXAMPLES**
High-order explosives (HE)	Produce a deafening supersonic overpressurization shock wave. Manufactured (military) explosives are exclusively HE based. May include improvised explosives. Terrorists may use HE or HE plus LE to create explosives.	TNT C-4 Semtex Nitroglycerin Dynamite Ammonium nitrate fuel oil (ANFO)
Low-order explosives (LE)	Create a subsonic explosion and lack HE's overpressurization wave. May include improvised explosives. Terrorists may use HE or HE plus LE to create explosives.	Pipe bombs Gunpowder Pure petroleum-based bombs

TABLE 8-2	Categories of Blast Injuries	
CATEGORY	**BODY PART AFFECTED**	**TYPES OF INJURIES**
Primary Unique to HE Results from impact of overpressurization wave with body surfaces	Gas-filled structures are most susceptible: Lungs GI tract Middle ear	Blast lung Tympanic membrane (TM) rupture and middle ear damage Abdominal hemorrhage and perforation Globe (eye) rupture Concussion (traumatic brain injury without physical signs of head injury)
Secondary Results from flying debris and bomb fragments	Any body part may be affected	Penetrating ballistic (fragmentation) or blunt injuries Eye penetration (can be occult)
Tertiary Results from individuals being thrown by blast wind	Any body part may be affected	Fracture and traumatic amputation Closed and open brain injury
Quaternary All other explosion injuries Includes exacerbation or complications of existing conditions	Any body part may be affected	Burns Crush injuries Closed and open brain injury Asthma, chronic obstructive pulmonary disease (COPD), or other breathing problems from dust, smoke, or toxic fumes Angina Hyperglycemia Hypertension

NURSING IMPLICATIONS

- Prepare to treat victims with severe blood loss, head injuries, shrapnel/impaling injuries, broken bones, and smoke/dust/particle inhalation.
- The timeline is high after detonation, but dependent on the number of people affected.
- Potential disruptions include public health infrastructure failure, healthcare system failure, healthcare facility failure, healthcare system overcapacity, healthcare facility overcapacity, healthcare system damage, healthcare facility damage, transportation system failure,

transportation system damage, interruption of utilities, interruption of supplies, unsafe environment, contaminated food, contaminated water, and staffing issues.

- Risk to self and family is medium with or without PPE.
- Personal safety precautions include: IN FIELD—respirator mask, eye protection, hard hat; OUT OF FIELD—universal precautions.
- Communicate with EMS, public safety, and public health authorities.
- Immediate health priorities: Extrication and life support, trauma triage, life-threatening/severe injuries to trauma center, not nearest hospital.
- Urgent health priorities: Spinal immobilization, wound dressings, IV fluids.
- Search and rescue priorities: Victims trapped in collapsed structures and under debris.

MOST COMMON CONDITIONS AND INJURIES

Table 8-3 shows the most common injuries and conditions associated with explosives and mass casualty events, organized by body system.

TABLE 8-3	Most Common Injuries and Conditions
SYSTEM	**INJURY OR CONDITION**
Auditory	TM rupture, ossicular disruption, cochlear damage, foreign body
Eye, orbit, face	Perforated globe, foreign body, air embolism, fractures
Respiratory	Blast lung, hemothorax, pneumothorax, pulmonary contusion and hemorrhage, arteriovenous (A-V) fistulas (source of air embolism), airway epithelial damage, aspiration pneumonitis, sepsis
Digestive	Bowel perforation, hemorrhage, ruptured liver or spleen, sepsis, mesenteric ischemia from air embolism
Circulatory	Cardiac contusion, myocardial infarction from air embolism, shock, vasovagal hypotension, peripheral vascular injury, air embolism–induced injury
CNS injury	Concussion, closed and open brain injury, stroke, spinal cord injury, air embolism–induced injury
Renal injury	Renal contusion, laceration, acute renal failure caused by rhabdomyolysis, hypotension, and hypovolemia
Extremity injury	Traumatic amputation, fractures, crush injuries, compartment syndrome, burns, cuts, lacerations, acute arterial occlusion, air embolism–induced injury

Explosives/Mass Casualty Events

PART

4

PRIORITIES IN DISASTER SITE MANAGEMENT

Personal Protective Equipment

CRITICAL INFO

- Know who is responsible in your organization for help with the proper use of personal protective equipment (PPE).
- Understand the levels of PPE and what level protection is needed for each type of event.
- Know where PPE is located in your organization.
- Understand how to properly don, adjust, wear, and remove and discard PPE.
- Understand how to maintain PPE properly.
- Understand the limitations of PPE in protecting you from injury.

OVERVIEW

In the midst of chemical, biological, or radiological disasters, nurses risk exposure to harmful and potentially deadly materials. Protecting both nurses and other healthcare providers against secondary contamination and exposure to the harmful substances is thus a priority.

When treating an exposed or potentially exposed patient, nurses should adhere to the guidelines for personal protective equipment of the Occupational Safety and Health Administration (OSHA). In the *Code of Federal Regulations* Section 1910, OSHA outlines the types of PPE that should be worn in various emergency situations. There are four different types of PPE, which provide different levels of protection. OSHA classifies these as levels A, B, C, and D.

The level of PPE required for nurses varies depending on the agent involved, the risk of exposure to the contaminant, and the assigned responsibilities of the nurse during the event.

IMPORTANT CONSIDERATIONS FOR WEARING PPE

Wearing PPE may present various problems for you depending on the environment, the level of PPE that is required, and the duration that the PPE will be worn. You should be prepared to expect any of the following conditions:

- Extreme heat
- Poor ventilation
- Lack of peripheral vision because of goggles or head gear
- Inhibited sense of touch because of gloves
- Claustrophobia
- Heavy weight

CAUTION

- If PPE does not fit properly, it will not be effective.
- Do not use respirators in a flammable or explosive atmosphere.
- Keep batteries/battery packs away from heat and flame.
- Know the proper procedure for donning and removing PPE.

It is important to determine if your hospital or agency has *enough* PPE in the event of a disaster and if any mitigation plans are in place in the event of an equipment shortage.

LEVELS OF PROTECTION

OSHA's four levels of protection against chemical substances—A, B, C, and D—are described in Table 9-1.

DONNING, DOFFING, AND ADJUSTING PPE

It is important to understand the proper technique for donning, removing, and adjusting PPE. If your role during a disaster or public health event will require wearing PPE, be sure you understand the appropriate procedures based on your organization's recommendations.

PROTECTION TYPES

Different protection is needed to protect the lungs, eyes, face, head, feet, and hands of nurses who respond to a disaster.

RESPIRATORY PROTECTION

Appropriate respiratory protection is a critical component for maintaining a safe working environment. Surgical masks offer no protection against chemical exposure. Therefore, depending on the type of chemical release, respirators may need to be worn. Respirators can be divided into two types: air-purifying and atmosphere-supplying.

1. Air-purifying respirators contain a filter element that removes contaminants from the air that is passing through it.
2. Atmosphere-supplying respirators use an air tank that supplies air to the breathing zone independent of the outside environment. They can be subdivided into self-contained breathing apparatus (SCBA) and positive pressure supplied-air respirators.

Advantages and disadvantages of each respirator type are discussed in Table 9-2.

Personal Protective Equipment

TABLE 9-1   OSHA's Level A, B, C, and D Protection Against Chemical Substances

LEVEL OF PROTECTION	EQUIPMENT	SHOULD BE USED WHEN
	A	
Highest available level of protection for: Respiratory Skin and eye Liquid splash Chemical vapors/gases	*Recommended:* Pressure-demand, full face piece self-contained breathing apparatus (SCBA) or pressure-demanded, supplied-air respirator (SAR) with escape SCBA Fully-encapsulated, vapor protective suit (meets National Fire Protection Association, 1991) Inner chemical-resistant gloves Chemical-resistant safety boots/shoes Two-way radio communication *Optional:* Cooling unit Hard hat Outer gloves and boot covers Two-way radio communication	The chemical substance has been identified and requires the highest level of protection for skin, eyes, and respiratory systems based on: Measured (or potential for) high concentration of atmospheric vapors, gases, or particulates; or Substances with high degree of hazard to skin are known or suspected to be present, and skin contact is possible Operations must be conducted in confined, poorly ventilated areas

B

Highest available level of protection for:
- Respiratory
- Eye

Less protection than level A for:
- Skin
- Liquid splash

No protection against:
- Chemical vapors/gases

Recommended:
- Pressure-demand, full face piece SCBA or pressure-demanded, SAR with escape SCBA
- Liquid splash protective suit (meets National Fire Protection Association, 1992)
- Inner chemical-resistant gloves
- Chemical-resistant safety boots/shoes
- Hard hat

Optional:
- Cooling unit
- Outer gloves and boot covers
- Two-way radio communication

The type and atmospheric concentration of substances have been identified and require high level of respiratory protection but less skin protection; this involves:

Atmosphere with an immediately dangerous to life and health (IDLH) concentration of specific substances that does not represent a severe skin hazard; or

Atmosphere containing less than 19.5% oxygen

Presence of incompletely identified vapors or gases (but not suspected of containing high levels of chemicals harmful to skin/capable of being absorbed through skin)

Level B is the minimum level recommended for initial site entries until the hazards have been identified

C

Same level of protection as level B for:
- Skin and eye

Less protection than level B for:
- Respiratory protection

No protection against:
- Liquid splash
- Chemical vapors/gases

Recommended:
- Full-face piece, air-purifying, canister-equipped respirator
- Support function protective garment (meets National Fire Protection Association, 1993)
- Chemical-resistant gloves and safety boots
- Two-way radio communication

Optional:
- Hard hat
- Escape SCBA
- Face shield

The atmosphere contains no known hazard

Work functions preclude splashes, immersion, or potential for unexpected inhalation or contact with hazardous levels of any chemical

NOTE: Not acceptable for chemical emergency response

Continued

TABLE 9-1	OSHA's Level A, B, C, and D Protection Against Chemical Substances—cont'd
LEVEL OF PROTECTION	**EQUIPMENT**	**SHOULD BE USED WHEN**

D

LEVEL OF PROTECTION	EQUIPMENT	SHOULD BE USED WHEN
Minimum protection for:	*Recommended:*	The atmosphere contains no known hazards
Skin and eye	Coveralls	Work functions preclude splashes, immersion, or
Liquid splash	Safety boots/shoes	potential for unexpected inhalation or contact with
No protection for:	Safety glasses or chemical splash goggles	hazardous levels of any chemical
Respiratory	*Optional:*	**NOTE:** Not acceptable for chemical emergency
Chemical vapors/gases	Gloves	response
	Escape SCBA	
	Face shield	

Modified from NIOSH/OSHA/USCG/EPA: *Occupational Safety and Health guidance manual for hazardous waste site activities*, Washington, DC, 1985, Department of Health and Human Services.

TABLE 9-2   Advantages and Disadvantages of Respirator Types

RESPIRATOR TYPE	ADVANTAGES	DISADVANTAGES
Air-Purifying	Enhanced mobility Lighter in weight than SCBA; weighs ≤2 pounds	Cannot be used in IDLH or oxygen-deficient atmosphere (<19.5% oxygen at sea level) Limited duration of protection; may be hard to gauge safe operating time in field conditions Only protects against specific chemicals and up to specific concentrations Use requires monitoring of contaminant and oxygen levels Can only be used: Against gas and vapor contaminants with adequate warning properties For specific gases or vapors, provided that service is known and safety factor is applied, or if unit has an end-of-service-life-indicator (ESLI)

Continued

TABLE 9-2   Advantages and Disadvantages of Respirator Types—cont'd

RESPIRATOR TYPE	ADVANTAGES	DISADVANTAGES
Atmosphere-Supplying		
SCBA	Provides highest available level of protection against airborne contaminants and oxygen deficiency Provides highest available level of protection under strenuous work conditions	Bulky, heavy (up to 35 pounds) Finite air supply limits work duration May impair movement in confined spaces
Positive pressure supplied-air respirator (SAR)	Enables longer work periods than SCBA Less bulky and heavy than SCBA; SAR equipment weighs <5 pounds (or ≈15 pounds, if escape SCBA protection is included) Protects against most airborne contaminants	Not approved for use in IDLH environments or oxygen-deficient atmospheres (<19.5% oxygen at sea level) unless equipped with an emergency egress unit, such as an escape-only SCBA, in case of air line failure Impairs mobility Mine Safety and Health Administration (MSHA)/National Institute for Occupational Safety and Health (NIOSH) certification limits hose length to 300 feet As length of hose is increased, minimum approved airflow may not be delivered at faceplate Air line is vulnerable to damage, chemical contamination, and degradation; decontamination of hoses may be difficult Worker must retrace steps to leave work area Requires supervision/monitoring of air supply line

EYE AND FACE PROTECTION

- Nurses must be provided with a sufficient number of goggles or face shields that provide maximum protection against such hazards as flying debris, gases, or liquids.
- Wearers of prescription lenses must be provided with eye protection that incorporates the prescription into its design or protection that can be worn over prescription lenses without disturbing the prescription of the eyewear.
- Contact lenses require that the wearer use proper eye and face protection and, because of the splash hazard, may be inappropriate for certain situations involving chemicals.
- Face shields should always be worn over primary eye protection, such as safety glasses or goggles, since they alone do not provide maximum protection.
- In instances when nurses may be exposed to chemicals or other corrosive materials, eyewash facilities meeting the requirements of American National Standard for Personal Protection (ANSI) Z358.1 should be established.
- Nurses should be equipped with ample supplies for emergency eye washes and should be prepared to conduct eye washes on self as well as on other responders.

HEAD PROTECTION

To prevent injuries to the head caused by falling objects, wear proper head protection.

FOOT PROTECTION

Proper foot protection must be worn to prevent exposure to infectious agents or toxic chemicals as well as to prevent physical injuries associated with emergency operations. Safety footwear should follow ANSI Z41. 1-1991 guidelines. Footwear should provide impact protection and be worn when carrying or handling anything that may fall. Footwear must furthermore provide puncture protection at scenes where sharp objects could fall and injure the foot. In certain instances, footwear should be equipped with steel toes and shanks, metatarsal protection, and oil- or skid-resistant soles, depending on the presenting hazards.

HAND PROTECTION

To protect nurses from chemicals, lacerations, abrasions, punctures, burns, biological agents, or temperature extremes, suitable gloves must be worn. No one type of glove is capable of protecting the wearer from all possible hazards; nurses must therefore choose the glove based on its performance characteristic relative to the hazards, the length of time that the glove is to be worn, and how likely the nurse would wear the glove. *In certain disaster incidents, the use of multiple gloves may be required.*

The use of gloves does not eliminate the need for hand hygiene. Likewise, the use of hand hygiene does not eliminate the need for gloves. The Centers for Disease Control and Prevention (CDC) recommends alcohol-based hand rubs be used before and after each patient just as gloves should be changed before and after each patient.

TRANSMISSION PRECAUTIONS

In the event of a bioterrorist attack, additional measures may be needed to augment standard nursing precautions. Depending upon the agent, airborne, droplet, or contact precautions may be required.

AIRBORNE PRECAUTIONS

Airborne transmission involves infected microorganisms or dust particles that remain suspended in the air for long periods of time and can be dispersed widely by air currents. Depending on environmental factors, a susceptible host may inhale particles within the same room or over a longer distance from the source patient.

Special air handling and ventilation are required to prevent airborne transmission.

In addition to standard precautions, airborne precautions include patient placement in a negative pressure room, use of respiratory protection such as an N95 respirator, and limitation of patient transport.

DROPLET PRECAUTIONS

Droplets can be transmitted from coughing, sneezing, and talking, and during certain procedures such as suctioning and bronchoscopy. Transmission is via the host's conjunctivae, nasal mucosa, or mouth.

Droplets do not remain suspended in the air and as such ventilation is not needed.

Do not confuse droplet transmission with airborne transmission.

In addition to standard precautions, droplet precautions include placement of the patient in a private room; use of a mask, especially when within three (3) feet of the patient; and limited patient transport.

CONTACT PRECAUTIONS

Contact transmission is the most frequent mode of transmission of nosocomial infections and is divided into the following two types:

1. *Direct-contact transmission.* Involves a body-to-body contact resulting in the physical transfer of microorganisms, such as bathing or turning a patient
2. *Indirect-contact transmission.* Involves a susceptible host touching a contaminated object (e.g., instruments, needles, dressings, doorknobs, etc.) or hands that are not washed and gloves that are not changed between patients

Gloves should always be used in contact precautions.

Gowns should be worn if there will be body-to-body contact or the patient has diarrhea, an ostomy, or excessive wound drainage.

Before leaving the patient's room, remove gloves and gown and thoroughly wash hands; be sure to avoid contact with any contaminated surfaces.

CHAPTER (10)

Triage

Triage

CRITICAL INFO

- Implement appropriate precautions when triaging potentially contaminated patients to avoid exposing yourself to the toxins or the physiological effects from wearing and working in personal protective gear.
- Be familiar with your facility's definitions and methods of triage in the disaster situations and understand how they differ from daily hospital triage.
- Understand the features of your facility's field triage tags and the triage color coding used therein—most prehospital disaster triage systems use the following color-coding system:
  - **RED** = Critical
  - **YELLOW** = Urgent
  - **GREEN** = Delayed
  - **BLACK** = Expectant: deceased or nonsalvageable
- Understand how your facility plans to triage those who are asymptomatic, those who might have been exposed, victims' family members, and the media, for example.

OVERVIEW

Triage is the process of prioritizing which patients are to be treated first and is the cornerstone of good disaster management. It is the first action in any disaster response, and decisions made at this time will have a significant impact upon the health outcomes of the affected population.

Disaster triage is a difficult and intimidating task. The presentation of multiple casualties can quickly overwhelm the facility and the healthcare personnel who must respond. Disaster triage in the field presents even greater challenges.

In a large-scale disaster or mass casualty incident, in all likelihood many healthcare providers will be called upon to perform triage at the scene or in the healthcare facility, including those without previous triage experience. In the hospital or at the scene, the triage nurse must accurately decide which patients need care, in what order they should receive care, and, in situations of severely constrained resources, who should not receive care at all.

In situations involving acute chemical exposures and hazardous materials (Hazmat) incidents, special conditions' triage must be employed. Decontamination should be performed whenever known or suspected contamination has occurred with a hazardous substance in either aerosol, solid, or liquid form. (Decontamination is discussed in depth in Chapter 11.)

Care must be taken to protect others from being secondarily exposed or further contamination of the environment.

TRIAGE CATEGORIES

One model for understanding triage consists of the following five conceptual categories:
1. Daily triage
2. Mass casualty incident (MCI) triage
3. Disaster triage
4. Tactical-military triage
5. Special conditions' triage

While all types of triage assign a priority to the order for receiving care, the determinants for priority of care differ. The five-category model for triage is shown in Table 10-1.

SUCCESSFUL DISASTER TRIAGE PRINCIPLES

The following successful disaster triage principles have been derived from historical experience:
1. Never move a casualty backward (against the flow).
2. Never hold a critical patient for further care.
3. Salvage life over limb.
4. Triage providers do not stop to treat patients.

Never move patients before triage except in the following cases: risks exist because of bad weather or impending or existing darkness; there is a continued risk of injury; medical facilities are immediately available; or a tactical situation dictates movement.

TRIAGE SYSTEMS

The following are three well-known triage systems:
- Simple triage and rapid treatment (START) system (for triaging adults)
- JumpSTART system (for triaging pediatric patients)
- Start/Save

SIMPLE TRIAGE AND RAPID TREATMENT (START) SYSTEM

The START system is a triage system used for prehospital triage. Emergency medical service (EMS) providers are normally the first responders to the scene of a disaster and are very experienced in triage and the START system.

TABLE 10-1   Five-Category Triage Model

TRIAGE CONCEPTUAL CATEGORY	SUMMARY/DESCRIPTION
1. Daily	Performed by nurses on a routine basis every day in the emergency department. The highest intensity of care is provided to the most seriously ill patients, even if they have a low probability of survival.
2. Mass casualty incident (MCI)	Emergency department is stressed by a large number of patients but remains functional; seriously ill still receive highest intensity of care. Additional resources are used but disaster plans have not been activated.
3. Disaster	Local emergency services are overwhelmed to the point that immediate care cannot be provided to everyone who needs it. "Do the greatest good for the greatest number." Identify injured patients who have a good chance of survival with immediate care. Four categories exist: lightly injured (can safely wait for care without risk), seriously injured, critically injured, and hopelessly injured.
4. Tactical-military	Military mission objectives rather than traditional nursing guidelines drive the triage and transport decisions.
5. Special conditions	Used when patients present from incidents involving weapons of mass destruction (WMD) such as radiation, biological, or chemical contaminants; mandate personal protective equipment (PPE) for all healthcare personnel, and decontamination capabilities at the facility.

The START system is easy to learn and simple to use. It is based on the respiratory system and mental status of the patient. All patients who can walk (walking wounded) are categorized as delayed (GREEN) and are asked to move away from the incident area to a specific location.

The next group of patients is assessed quickly (30 to 60 seconds per patient) by evaluating RPM:

- Respiration (position upper airway or determine respiratory rate)
- Perfusion/blood circulation (check capillary refill time)
- Mental status (determine patient's ability to obey commands)

The RPM components are assessed in order. For example, if the victim is not breathing, CPR is not performed—the patient is categorized as expectant (BLACK) and the assessor moves on to the next victim.

Table 10-2 summarizes the classifications based upon the patient's RPM findings.

Victims are tagged with a corresponding colored triage tag, provided with basic field care for stabilization, and transported in order of priority. When a patient arrives at an emergency department (ED) with a tag, the ED triage team must still triage the patient, as the condition may have changed during transport.

JUMPSTART

Because the physiological indicators used in START are not appropriate when assessing young pediatric patients, the JumpSTART system was created to meet the unique needs of assessing children less than eight (8) years of age. Because it may be difficult to determine actual age during a disaster, JumpSTART should be used if the victim "looks like a child" and START used if the victim "looks like a young adult or older."

NOTE: JumpSTART was designed for use in disaster/multicasualty settings and *not* for daily EMS or hospital triage. JumpSTART is also intended for the triage of children with acute injuries and may not be appropriate for primary triage of children with medical illnesses in a disaster setting.

In this triage system a child's respiratory rate is assessed as "good" if it is between 15 and 45 breaths per minute (approximately 1 breath every 2 to 4 seconds). A child with a rate less than 15 or greater than 45 breaths per minute would be classified as critical (RED).

A child's perfusion is checked by palpating the distal pulses. A child with a weak or non-existent distal pulse is classified as critical (RED).

TABLE 10-2 Using RPM to Classify Patients	
CATEGORY (COLOR)	**RPM INDICATORS**
Critical (RED)	R = Respiratory rate >30/minute P = Capillary refill >2 seconds M = Does not obey commands
Urgent (YELLOW)	R <30/minute P <2 seconds M = Obeys commands
Expectant: dead or dying (BLACK)	R = Not breathing

Assess for mental status using the AVPU system: Alert, responds to Vocal stimuli, responds to Painful stimuli, Unresponsive. A child who is unresponsive or who gives an inappropriate response to pain would be classified as critical (RED).

In addition, unlike the START system, in the JumpSTART system a young child who is not breathing on initial assessment should still be checked for a pulse. If a pulse is found, the child receives a brief (5 breaths) ventilatory trial that if unsuccessful results in assigning the patient as expectant (BLACK). If breathing is restored, the patient is classified as critical (RED).

For additional information on JumpSTART, refer to www. jumpstarttriage.com.

START/SAVE TRIAGE FOR CATASTROPHIC DISASTERS

Some disaster events are of such magnitude and duration that rapid evacuation of the victims is not possible. Occasionally an event occurs that requires that victims be evaluated immediately, but because of the inability to evacuate the patient to a higher source of care, the triage process must be extended.

The Medical Disaster Response (MDR) project was developed to specifically address an event where specially trained local healthcare providers evaluate patients immediately after the event, but cannot evacuate patients to definitive care. In this type of scenario, a dynamic triage methodology was developed that permits the triage process to evolve over hours or even days, thereby maximizing patient survival and resulting in a more efficient use of resources. This MDR system incorporates a modified version of simple triage and rapid treatment (START) that substitutes radial pulse for capillary refill, coupled with a system of secondary triage termed secondary assessment of victim endpoint (SAVE) (Benson, Koenig, and Schultz, 1996).

The SAVE triage was developed to direct limited resources to the subgroup of patients expected to benefit most from their use. SAVE assesses survivability of patients with various injuries and, on the basis of trauma statistics, uses this information to describe the relationship between expected benefits and resources consumed. Because early transport to an intact medical system is unavailable, this information guides treatment priorities in the field to a level beyond the scope of the START methodology.

Pre-existing disease and age are factored into the triage decisions. For example, an elderly patient with burns to 70% of the body surface area who is unsalvageable under austere conditions and would require the use of significant medical resources (both personnel and equipment) would be triaged to an "expectant area." Conversely, a young adult with a Glasgow coma scale score of 12 who requires only airway maintenance would use few resources and would have a reasonable chance fur survival with the interventions available in the field, and would be triaged to a "treatment area."

The START and SAVE triage techniques are used in situations in which triage is dynamic and occurs over many hours to days, and only limited, austere, field, advanced life support equipment is readily available.

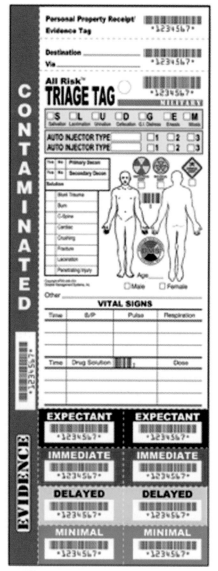

Figure 10-1. Sample triage tag.

TRIAGE TAGS

Many different types of triage tag systems are available. Tags are designed to be attached to a patient's arm or leg—not their clothing—and should contain as much information about the patient as is possible (e.g., name, triage number, triage category, decontamination status, presenting injury/complaint, interventions performed, date/time, allergies, medication history, etc.).

Some triage tags have perforated colored tabs for the different triage classifications, so if the patient's condition changes and deteriorates, the tag may be torn again to the revised triage level/color (Figure 10-1). Others are all one color (red, yellow, green, or black), and some include contamination or decontamination information.

All tags must be waterproof, easy to write on, easy to read, and clearly visible when attached to the patient.

TRIAGE FOR CHEMICAL/HAZARDOUS MATERIALS DISASTERS

Disasters involving chemicals or hazardous materials pose a threat to the safety and health of care providers. Nurses need to implement certain

TABLE 10-3	Three Zones of Disaster Triage and Decontamination*
ZONE	**DESCRIPTION OF ACTIVITIES**
Hot	Immediately adjacent to location of incident
	Minimal triage and medical care; activities are limited to airway and hemorrhage control, administration of antidotes, and identification of expectant cases
	All staff are in protective gear in this zone
Warm	More than 300 feet from outer edge of hot zone, and uphill/upwind from contamination area
	Rapid triage takes place to sort victims into critical, urgent, delayed, or expectant categories
	Priority is to commence decontamination
	All staff must wear appropriate PPE
Cold	Adjacent to warm zone, and uphill/upwind from contamination area
	Decontaminated patients enter this area where a more thorough triage is performed; then patients are directed to treatment areas based upon severity and nature of illness or injury
	Personnel may wear PPE in case the wind changes or victims arrive who have been improperly decontaminated

*Further information on decontamination may be found in Chapter 11.

precautions when providing care and treating potentially contaminated patients to avoid exposing themselves to the toxins or the physiological effects from wearing and working in personal protective gear. In addition, victims who are chemically contaminated must be decontaminated before being brought into a clean treatment area.

Since treatment of patients initially begins at the site of the incident, specific procedures for decontamination should thus be implemented in the field. However, the walking wounded may leave the scene before triage and decontamination and may need to be decontaminated upon arrival at a treatment facility.

TRIAGE AND DECONTAMINATION ZONES

Emergency responders should immediately establish the following three zones for triage, some medical care activities, and decontamination:

1. Hot zone
2. Warm zone
3. Cold zone

Table 10-3 describes the activities in each of the three zones.

CHAPTER 11

Decontamination

CRITICAL INFO

- Review your organization's/agency's Incident Command System (ICS), Hospital Incident Command System HICS (if relevant), and triage/decontamination methods as well as the availability of recommended personal protective equipment (PPE), if your role will involve decontamination or interaction with potentially contaminated victims.
- Decontaminate patients as soon as possible.
- Disrobing is decontamination; head to toe—the more clothing that is removed, the better; 90% of contaminants can be removed by disrobing.
- Thorough decontamination is desired since incompletely decontaminated patients may contaminate healthcare workers.
- Be sure to label patients with their current decontamination status.
- Keep children and parent(s) or older siblings together if possible during decontamination.
- Once an individual enters a decontamination or contaminated area, they and their PPE/equipment require decontamination before entering the clean treatment area. For large-scale incidents, exit and entrance to the scene/facility must be tightly controlled.
- Wet babies are slippery!
- Children will be afraid.

OVERVIEW

Decontamination removes (or reduces) contaminating agent(s) from victims while keeping staff and others protected from being secondarily exposed and preventing further contamination of the environment. It must be available and provided quickly to patients whenever a known or suspected contamination has occurred through contact with an aerosol, solid, or liquid hazardous substance. Management and treatment of contaminated victims vary depending upon the situation and the nature of the hazardous substance. There are two types of decontamination:

- Technical (equipment and personnel)
- Medical/patient (injured or exposed individuals)

Technical decontamination is a regimented method used by hazardous materials' teams that often uses solutions to better clean or neutralize a chemical product. Medical or patient decontamination is usually performed by first responders on-scene or by first receivers in the hospital setting.

The first consideration for disasters involving chemicals or hazardous materials is staff safety. Nurses need to implement certain precautions when providing care and treating potentially contaminated patients to avoid exposing themselves to the toxins or the physiological effects from wearing and working in personal protective gear. Take care to ensure you are wearing the appropriate PPE for the job you are assigned. (See Chapter 9 to learn more about the various types of PPE, the protection they provide, and their impact on you physiologically.)

Since treatment of patients may initially begin at the site of the incident, decontamination may be implemented on-scene and/or in the hospital setting. You should be familiar with the work zones in either setting. These are discussed in further detail later in this chapter.

The following are essential requirements for any decontamination task:

- A safe area to keep a patient while undergoing decontamination
- A method for washing contaminants off a patient
- A means of containing the rinsate (control runoff)
- Adequate protection for personnel treating the patient; the PPE used by decontamination personnel should be no less than one level below that used for entry into the hazardous environment
- Disposable or cleanable medical equipment to treat patients

WORK ZONES

Controlling the site during decontamination, whether on-scene or at the hospital, is critical to reducing the accidental spread of the contaminant by victims, responders/staff, or equipment.

By dividing the site into work zones, triage and decontamination work activities can be confined to appropriate areas to minimize the risk of accidental exposures. Zones also assist in locating and evacuating personnel in the event of an emergency and, when well controlled, prevent unauthorized persons from entering.

Work zones vary depending on the nature of the release and the location:

- On-scene
- Hospital-based

ON-SCENE WORK ZONES

When responders establish a perimeter after estimating potential hazards and response activities, the area should have the following characteristics:

- Be uphill and upwind from the contaminated area
- Be based on the topography and possible access routes to the area

- Be larger than necessary since it is easier to shrink an area than it is to expand it
- Encompass additional zones (work zones) within it to allow for easier patient triage, decontamination, and treatment

Although an on-scene site may be divided into as many zones as necessary to ensure minimal exposure of responders to hazardous substances, the three most frequently identified zones are as follows (Table 11-1):

1. Exclusion (or hot zone)
2. Contamination reduction (or warm zone)
3. Support (clean zone or cold zone)

HOSPITAL SETTING WORK ZONES

In the event of a chemical or hazardous material release, hospitals and other healthcare facilities also need to establish work zones (Table 11-2). These are generally referred to as follows:

- Hot
- Warm (dirty)
- Cold (clean)

TECHNICAL DECONTAMINATION

For both on-scene and hospital setting decontamination, there may also be a technical decontamination zone (for decontaminating PPE and equipment).

DECONTAMINATION PRIORITIZATION

In the hot zone, when resources are limited and the number of victims is high, responders may have to prioritize patients for receiving decontamination, treatment, and medical evaluation while providing *the greatest benefit for the greatest number with the least amount of harm.*

Determining where to treat and whether to treat or decontaminate a nonambulatory patient who is symptomatic is a particularly difficult part of this prioritization/triage. There should be protocols established by your local emergency response agencies based on the nature of the release, the amount of antidote or post-exposure vaccine available, and the number of workers available to transport and treat large numbers of victims.

After sorting victims into ambulatory and nonambulatory, the general guidelines in Table 11-3 may be useful for ambulatory patients.

Nonambulatory patients (unconscious, unresponsive, unable to move unassisted) remain in place while further prioritization for decontamination occurs. Recommended guidelines, which follow the prioritization (color-coding system) used in the medical triage system called START (simple triage and rapid treatment system), are outlined in Table 11-4.

TABLE 11-1	On-Scene Decontamination Work Zones

ZONE	DESCRIPTION
Exclusion/hot	Is a contaminated area or area with greatest potential for exposure. All personnel entering this area must wear appropriate level of PPE for degree and types of hazards. Outer boundary, or hotline, separates area of contamination from contamination reduction zone, either with a physical barrier (such as fence, rope, hazard tape) or with signs. Along periphery of this zone, access control points may be established to control personnel and equipment entering and leaving contaminated area. In some cases this zone may be subdivided further, depending upon contaminant and other factors. Some of these subdivisions may include ambulatory patient assembly areas, and triage and secondary triage areas (for both ambulatory and nonambulatory victims).
Contamination reduction/ warm	Is a decontamination area. All personnel entering this area must wear PPE no more than one level below PPE worn in exclusion zone. Contamination control line separates this zone from exclusion and support zones. Access control points for this zone are to ensure that personnel are wearing proper PPE to enter exclusion zone and that personnel exiting contamination reduction zone to support zone remove or decontaminate all potentially contaminated PPE. Personnel, ambulatory and nonambulatory patients and equipment are decontaminated in designated areas within this zone in an area referred to as contamination-reduction corridor.
Support/clean/ cold	Is an uncontaminated area. No PPE is required in this area, since personnel are unlikely to become contaminated in this zone. Any potentially contaminated clothing, equipment, and samples (outer containers) should not be permitted in this zone. Command post supervisor as well as administrative, medical, and support personnel (to help keep other zones running) set up work areas in this zone. These may include an entry PPE layout area, a clean patient treatment area, a rapid treatment area, and access to transportation to healthcare facilities and/or shelters.

Decontamination

Decontamination

TABLE 11-2   Hospital Decontamination Work Zones

ZONE	LOCATION	DESCRIPTION
Hot	Contamination site (prehospital)	Is a contaminated area where release occurred. See discussion of on-scene decontamination (see Table 11-1).
Warm/dirty	Adjacent to hospital, usually near emergency department (remote to release site)	Is a hospital decontamination area. This area needs a source of water (cold climates require a warm water source) for decontamination and barriers to control entrance and exit from area, which must be tightly controlled. Personnel working in this area (first receivers) have potential to be exposed to contaminant(s), and therefore must wear appropriate level of PPE (level C minimum). At entrance to the warm zone is the initial triage station. All ambulance and walk-in cases must enter facility after going through this triage station. Victims who are clearly not contaminated skip the warm zone and enter the cold (clean) zone directly. All others proceed into the warm zone for decontamination.
Cold/clean	Hospital treatment area, often emergency department	Is an uncontaminated hospital treatment area (postdecontamination). Since no agent exposure is expected in this area, in most cases only standard (universal) precautions are needed for healthcare workers. This area needs to be tightly controlled so that only patients that have been triaged and decontaminated are allowed entry. Any potentially contaminated victims, clothing, PPE, and/or equipment should not be permitted to enter this zone. Another more thorough triage is performed in cold (clean) zone before treatment is begun based on nature and acuity of signs and symptoms.

DECONTAMINATION PRIORITY	AMBULATORY PATIENT CRITERIA
First priority: Direct to warm zone for immediate decontamination	• Closest to point of release • Report exposure to an aerosol/mist or have known liquid agent contamination serious signs/symptoms (e.g., dyspnea, chest tightness, etc.)
Second priority	• Not as close to point of release • May or may not have known liquid agent contamination, but patients are clinically symptomatic (moderate to minimal signs/symptoms)
Third priority	• Suffering from conventional injuries (e.g., open wounds)
Lowest priority: Direct to ambulatory assembly area in warm zone for further review	• Far from point of release • No known/suspected exposure to liquid, aerosol, or vapor • Minimal or no signs/symptoms

TABLE 11-3   Ambulatory Patient Decontamination Prioritization

Decontamination

A note regarding on-scene decontamination: There may be extreme cases where victims in the hot zone must be treated before decontamination (e.g., airway maintenance, antidote administration). The most effective initial decontamination of these patients in the hot zone is clothing removal, followed by more thorough decontamination in the warm zone, if appropriate.

METHODS

There are two basic methods for decontamination:
1. Physical removal
2. Chemical deactivation
A more detailed description of each method appears in Table 11-5.

SUPPLIES

Proper equipment and supplies are needed to care for patients in each of the three decontamination zones. Typically it is the responsibility of the local fire department or hazardous materials (Hazmat) team to bring decontamination equipment to the scene of a disaster; find out who is responsible in your local area. The equipment and supplies listed in Table 11-6 are the minimum necessary to undertake decontamination procedures.

TABLE 11-4　Nonambulatory Patient Decontamination Prioritization and Relation to START Triage System

START CATEGORY	DECON PRIORITY	START MEDICAL CRITERIA	CONTAMINATION CRITERIA
RED (Critical)	1	Respiration present only after repositioning airway RPM: *Respiration:* respiratory rate >30/min *Perfusion:* capillary refill >2 sec *Mental status:* unable to obey commands	Closest to point of release Serious signs and symptoms and/or known liquid agent contamination or severe exposure
YELLOW (Urgent)	2	Injuries treatable or controllable on-scene for limited time RPM: *Respiration:* respiratory rate <30/min *Perfusion:* capillary refill <2 sec *Mental status:* able to obey commands	Close to point of release Moderate to minimal signs/symptoms and/or known/suspected liquid agent contamination or known aerosol contamination second priority
GREEN (Delayed)	3	Ambulatory Injuries do not require immediate treatment	Minimal signs/symptoms No known or suspected exposure to liquid, aerosol, or vapor
BLACK (Expectant: dead or non-salvageable)	4	Respiratory arrest, even after attempt to reposition airway	Severe signs/symptoms Grossly contaminated with liquid nerve agent Unresponsive to atropine injections

TABLE 11-5	Decontamination Methods

METHOD	DESCRIPTION
Physical removal	• **Remove clothing**—Clothing removal is decontamination; encourage victims to remove clothing at least to their undergarments. • **Flush** with water or aqueous solutions. • **Absorb** contaminating agent with absorbent materials (e.g., rub with flour followed by wet tissues or use military M291 resin kits for spot decontamination of skin only). • **Scrape** bulk agent with a wooden stick (e.g., tongue depressor/popsicle stick). • **NOTE:** Follow all of the above with full decontamination at a medical treatment facility.
Chemical deactivation	• **Water/soap wash:** Chemical warfare agents have a generally low solubility and slow rate of diffusion in both fresh water and seawater. Therefore the major effect of water and water combined with soap (especially with alkaline soaps) is via a slow breakdown of the compound (i.e., hydrolysis) or through dilution of the agent and the mechanical force of the wash. When other chemical deactivation means are not available, washing with water or with soap and water is a good alternative. • **Chemical solutions:** In the event of an emergency you may be directed to perform decontamination with other chemical deactivation agents. These vary depending upon the chemical warfare agent, and may include alkaline solutions of hypochlorite.

CATEGORIES OF DECONTAMINATION

Medical or patient decontamination may be divided into the following three categories:

• Individual patient decontamination
• Group (mass) decontamination
• Self-decontamination

The subcategories for each are outlined in Table 11-7.

Methods for Individual Decontamination

A description of decontamination procedures for each of the four subcategories of individual decontamination (gross, secondary, nonambulatory, and pediatric) is provided on the following pages.

TABLE 11-6   Decontamination Supplies and Equipment

BASELINE ITEMS NEEDED FOR DECONTAMINATION

- Containment equipment
- Pool or tank
- Tarps
- 6-mil construction plastic
- Fiberglass backboards
- Supports for ambulatory patients
- Sawhorses to support backboards
- Water supply
- Scissors for clothing removal
- Mild detergent (dishwashing liquid)
- Five-gallon buckets
- Sponges and soft brushes
- Towels and blankets/sheets
- Triage tags
- Disposable clothes and shoes for ambulatory patients
- Large plastic bags for contaminated clothing with predetermined unique ID tags to go on bag and patient's wrist/neck
- Small plastic bags for patients' valuables
- Waterproof pens to mark bags
- Clear, zip-front body suits or large water-repellant blankets to minimize contamination to transport personnel and ambulances
- Tape (duct, 4-inch)

TABLE 11-7   Subcategories of Decontamination

INDIVIDUAL DECONTAMINATION	GROUP DECONTAMINATION	SELF-DECONTAMINATION
• Gross patient decon • Secondary or definitive • Nonambulatory patients • Pediatric	• Mass population	• Personal • PPE

Individual decontamination may be divided into two steps:
1. Gross
2. Secondary (definitive)

Gross decontamination (Box 11-1) is the first step of the individual decontamination process. In this step, priority is given to airway, breathing, and circulation (ABC) and victims are flushed with massive amounts of water. This step generally removes the majority of contaminants. In the second step (secondary or definitive decontamination) (Box 11-2), victims are more thoroughly decontaminated using both soap and water in a systematic fashion to remove any residual contamination before being transferred to the support zone (for on-scene decontamination) or the cold (clean) zone (when in a hospital setting).

Nurses must wear appropriate PPE for both steps and until the threat of secondary exposure no longer exists.

BOX 11-1   Procedures for Gross Individual Patient Decontamination

- Direct patient to the decontamination area (warm zone).
- Separate male and female patients if possible, and keep children with parents or older sibling, if possible.
- Instruct patients to wipe feet before entering decontamination area— use mat or remove shoes directly into plastic bag.
- Instruct patient to remove clothing.
- Place clothing in plastic bag with shoes, label the bag, and hold it during decontamination.
- Instruct patient to place valuables in a small plastic bag, label the bag, and hold it during decontamination.
- Brush or wipe off particulate matter.
- Instruct patient to step into shower, close eyes and mouth, and raise arms above head.
- Instruct patient to rotate twice, slowly.
- Instruct patient to walk out of shower into secondary (definitive) decontamination area.

Nonambulatory Patients

Patients who cannot assist in their own decontamination present challenges to rescue workers (Box 11-3). When attending to nonambulatory patients, as with ambulatory patients, nurses should always wear appropriate PPE until the threat of secondary exposure no longer exists.

Pediatric Patients

When dealing with children in a disaster situation, nurses not only must work to identify, triage, and decontaminate a potentially large number of children, but also must take special precautions to ensure that the emotional and psychological trauma experienced by the children is minimized (Box 11-4).

Although decontamination always takes precedence, where possible, contain all runoff from decontamination procedures for proper disposal.

Methods for Group Decontamination

In a disaster involving a large number of patients, nurses will find it necessary to implement appropriate disaster triage protocols to prioritize patients' entry through the decontamination process. The decontamination procedures for a mass population incident are shown in Box 11-5.

BOX 11-2   Procedures for Secondary (Definitive) Individual Patient Decontamination

- If possible keep male and female patients separate.
- Make sure all clothing is removed, bagged, and labeled.
- Brush or vacuum any remaining particulate matter off of skin.
- Decontaminate systematically from the head down with water.
- Water-wash contaminated area gently under a stream of water and scrub gently using a soft brush with soap.
- Use warm, never hot, water.
- Decontaminate exposed wounds and eyes before intact skin areas; do not introduce contaminants into wounds.
- Cover wounds with a waterproof dressing.
- Remember the back, under skin folds, axilla, ears, and genitalia.
- Remove contaminants to the level that they are no longer a threat to the patient or response personnel.
- Allow ambulatory patients to decontaminate themselves.
- Provide instructions in multiple languages to ensure that patients understand the problem and follow instructions.
- Administer medicines or ventilation support to seriously ill patients while undergoing decontamination.
- Conduct invasive procedures in the contamination reduction zone (on-scene) or warm zone (hospital setting) only when it is absolutely necessary.
- Isolate the patient from the environment by wrapping in blanket/sheet to prevent the spread of any remaining contaminants.
- Direct men and women to segregated treatment areas, if possible.
- Soap, brushes, sponges, and other equipment used for decontamination should be placed in a trash can and not carried into the support zone (on-scene) or the cold (clean) zone (hospital setting).

BOX 11-3   Procedures for Individual Nonambulatory Patient Decontamination

- Apply C-collar immediately if a cervical spine injury is suspected.
- Place plastic sheet on cart, cover with sheet, place victim on sheet.
- Remove all clothing and place in plastic bag and label the bag.
- Place valuables in small plastic bag and label properly.
- Brush or wipe off particulate matter.
- Rinse patient gently using hand-held sprayer; begin with face and airway, then open wounds (cover patient's mouth and pinch nose when washing face).
- Ensure axilla, genitalia, and the back are rinsed.
- Use non-rebreather mask or bag-valve mask to protect airway.
- Wash from head to toe using tepid, not hot, water and soap five (5) minutes when agent is nonpersistent and eight (8) minutes when a persistent or unknown agent.
- Wash and rinse creases such as ears, eyes, axilla, groin; rinse for about 1 minute; roll patient to side if needed.
- Thoroughly dry patient and cover with a blanket.
- Soap, brushes, sponges, and other equipment used for decontamination should be placed in a trash can and not carried into the support zone (on-scene) or the cold (clean) zone (hospital setting).
- Open wounds should be covered with dressings after decontamination is complete.
- Transfer patient to clean backboard and exit into cold zone for rapid assessment, triage, and assignment to a treatment area.

BOX 11-4   Considerations for Pediatric Patient Decontamination

- Allow children and parents (or other adults known to them) to remain together.
- Constantly reassure and offer compassion to a child if the child is separated from his or her parent(s)—children will be fearful.
- Attempt to reunite children with their parents if they were separated during the course of the disaster.
- Take time to inform and reassure older children of the current situation.
- Prevent children from developing hypothermia.
- Use a water temperature of 100° F.
- Wash/shower for 5 minutes.
- Use great caution: wet infants are slippery.

BOX 11-5   Procedures for Mass Population Decontamination

- Use large volumes of water from charged hose lines to quickly rinse large numbers of individuals.
- Portable trailers and/or aerial ladder trucks with special spray systems containing both soap and water should be available.
- Have towels and temporary clothing for patients once the decontamination procedures are completed.
- Although decontamination always takes precedence, contain all runoff from decontamination procedures for proper disposal.

BOX 11-6   Procedures for Self-Decontamination

- Walk through gross decontamination shower wearing PPE, rotating twice.
- Enter technical decontamination area and dry PPE; then:
  - Remove tape (if used), securing gloves and boots to suit.
  - Remove outer gloves (if wearing inner gloves) while turning inside out.
  - Remove suit, turning it inside out and folding downward as it is removed.
  - Remove boots one at a time (do not place clean feet on wet/contaminated surface).
  - Remove mask/respirator, place in plastic bag, and hand to suit support.
  - Remove inner gloves and throw away within contaminated area.
  - Move to shower area, remove clothing, place in plastic bag, and shower.
- Proceed to rehabilitation area, weigh in, vital signs, rehydration.

Method for Self-Decontamination

Following the decontamination process, nurses will need to decontaminate themselves and their equipment before leaving the disaster scene to minimize the risk of cross-contamination. The procedure for self-decontamination may vary depending upon the contaminant, but in general expect the procedures shown in Box 11-6.

PART

5

CLINICAL MANAGEMENT

CHAPTER (12)

Burn Management

CRITICAL INFO

- Contact the National Center for Injury Prevention and Control at 1-770-488-1506 for more information about burns.
- Contact the American Burn Association at 1-800-548-2876 for more information about burns.
- Treating a burn in the first few minutes can impact the severity of the injury.
- Remove all burned clothing from the patient immediately; if clothing adheres to the skin, cut or tear around burned area.
- Remove all jewelry, belts, and tight clothing from over the burned areas and from around the victim's neck since burned areas swell quickly.

Burn
Management

OVERVIEW

Mass trauma incidents and disasters such as explosions and fires can cause a variety of serious injuries, including burns. A mass burn casualty disaster is defined by the American Burn Association as "any catastrophic event in which the number of burn victims exceeds the capacity of the local burn center to provide optimal burn care" (Saffle, Gibran, & Jordan, 2005). Burn injuries are common in mass casualty events and terrorist attacks; in most traumatic events, approximately 25% of those injured will require burn care. In the 2001 World Trade Center attacks, approximately one third of those hospitalized required burn care. Injuries include thermal burns, which are caused by contact with flames, hot liquids, hot surfaces, and other sources of high heat, as well as chemical, electrical, and toxic burns. Immediate care in the event of a burn not only is desirable but also is critical to saving lives.

NURSING ESSENTIALS OF ASSESSMENT AND MANAGEMENT OF THE BURN PATIENT

Evaluate all burn patients first as trauma patients.
- STOP the burning process
- Primary survey: adhere to ABCDEs
  - **A**irway management with C-spine control
  - Restore **B**reathing
  - Restore **C**irculation and **C**ontrol hemorrhage
  - Assess **D**isability
  - **E**xpose patient and control **E**nvironment

- Secondary survey
  - Identify the extent and depth of the burn
  - Identify the presence of inhalation injury, which is determined by meeting one or more of the following conditions:
    History of exposure to hot gases, steam, or combustible products
    Singed vibrissae and carbonaceous sputum
    Carbonaceous endobronchial debris or mucosal ulceration
    Abnormal xenon or technetium scan or elevated carboxyhemoglobin or cyanide levels
    Presence of circumferential burn wound component on the torso or extremities
    Presence of burns on the face, eyes, ears, hands, genitals, or feet
    Presence of electrical or chemical burns
    Presence or suspicion of abusive injury
  - Monitor extremities for compartment syndrome (REMOVE)
    Remove jewelry, constricting clothing
    Elevate extremity
    Motion (active range)
    Ongoing
    Vascular
    Exams and **E**scharotomy

DEFINITIVE CARE PHASE

Determine if components of the secondary survey constitute immediate management of the burns or transfer. This includes the following:
- Wound size is estimated by total body surface area (TBSA).
- Burn depth is determined by the physician.
- Intubate patients with severe facial burns or inhalation injury.
- Initiate fluid resuscitation based on time of injury and titrate to urine output.
- The essentials of wound care include cleanliness, moisture, and protection.
- Topical antimicrobials are reserved for deeper burns.
- Early nutrition and rapid increases to goal requirements are essential; ensure that tetanus immunization is up to date.
- Complications are common and predictable.

RULE OF NINES

To calculate the TBSA involved in burns, a method called the "rule of nines" is used. According to the rule of nines, the body is divided into sections and each specific area is assigned a value of 9 or 18, depending on its approximate percentage of the body surface area. The values that are assigned are as follows: head and neck, 9%; anterior thorax, 18%; posterior thorax, 18%; arms, 9% each; legs, 18% each; perineum, 1% (Figure 12-1).

RULE OF 1'S

The rule of 1's calculates a burn size score (BSS). Under this rule the head, anterior torso, posterior torso, genitals, each arm, and each leg are worth 1 point. If the area is burned >50%, a 1 is assigned. If the area is burned <50%, a 0.5 is assigned. The points are added and rounded up. For example, a man with burns to the head, anterior chest, and bilateral arms has a BSS of 4. To calculate the amount of intravenous (IV) lactated Ringer's (LR) needed per hour, use the following formula: 2.25 × BSS × weight (kg).

TRIAGE CATEGORIES

See Table 12-1 for triage categories, including priority, definition, and criteria. The following burns require referral to a burn unit:
- Partial thickness burns greater than 10% of TBSA
- Face, hands, feet, genitalia, perineum, or major joint burns
- Third-degree burns in any age group
- Electrical and chemical burns

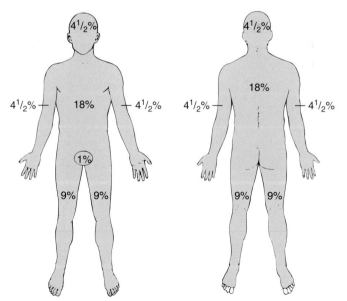

Figure 12-1. Rule of nines. *Left,* Anterior view. *Right,* Posterior view.

Burn Management

- Inhalation injury
- Burns in patients with a pre-existing condition that could affect recovery
- Burns in patients with concomitant trauma (e.g., fractures)
- Burns in children receiving care in a hospital without adequate equipment or personnel to care for children
- Burns in patients who require social, emotional, or long-term rehabilitative intervention

THERMAL INJURY MANAGEMENT

A thermal injury can result from a flame or steam and can cause denaturation of body proteins. This process breaks down the functions of the skin, such as regulating both bodily fluids and temperature, and maintaining a

TABLE 12-1   Triage Categories

PRIORITY	COLOR	DEFINITION	CRITERIA
1	Red	Critically injured patients who require immediate care and treatment at a burn center	• TBSA >60%, with or without injury, inhalation injury • TBSA 40%-60% with inhalation injury • Infant TBSA >10% or children TBSA >15% • Any pediatric patient with inhalation injury
2	Yellow	Urgent patients who require treatment at a burn center	• TBSA 20%-60% and no inhalation injury • TBSA 0%-40% with inhalation injury • Infant TBSA <10% or children TBSA <15%
3	Green	Patients who do not meet American Burn Association criteria for treatment at a burn center	• TBSA 0%-20% and no inhalation injury
4	Black	Patients with a poor prognosis for survival	• Deceased or cardiac arrest • Patients with all burns >40%, age >60 years, and inhalation injury

protective barrier against foreign pathogens. Burns are further classified into first-degree, second-degree, and third-degree burns depending on the extent of their severity. The severity of a thermal injury is determined by the following:

- The temperature of the agent
- The length of exposure to the agent
- The thickness of the area exposed
- Depth and extent (%TBSA) of the burn
- Age
- Presence of smoke inhalation

FIRST-DEGREE BURNS

First-degree burns involve the outermost layer of the skin (epidermis). Sunburn is an example of a first-degree burn.

Signs
- Red
- Painful
- Hyperemic
- Skin will show mild swelling
- Damage only to epidermis
- Complete scarless healing in 7 days

Medical Management for Nurses

Do's
- Apply cool, wet compresses to the affected area until pain subsides.
- Cover the burn with a sterile, nonadhesive bandage or clean cloth.
- To help alleviate pain and discomfort, patients may use over-the-counter pain medications.
- First-degree burns usually heal without further treatment; however, if a first-degree burn covers a large area of the body, or the victim is an infant or elderly, seek emergency medical attention.

Don'ts
- Do not apply topical medication to burn.
- Do not apply ice.
- Do not open the blisters.

SECOND-DEGREE BURNS

Second-degree burns involve the first two layers of the skin (epidermis and dermis).

Superficial Second-Degree Burns

Signs
- Damage to epidermis and some dermis
- Very painful
- Blisters
- Heals in 2 weeks with minimal scarring

Deep Second-Degree Burns

Signs
- Damage to epidermis and most dermis
- Relatively insensate
- No blisters/white waxy, moist appearance
- Heals in many weeks with hypertrophic scar

Medical Management for Nurses

Do's
- Immerse in fresh, cool water or apply a cold, wet compress for 10-15 minutes.
- Dry with clean cloth and cover with sterile gauze.
- Elevate burned arms or legs.
- Take steps to prevent shock: lay the victim flat; elevate burned arms and legs about 12 inches.
- In chemical burns, remove or dilute the chemical agent with water.
- Contact the nearest hospital or tertiary medical center that is equipped to handle second-degree burns.

Don'ts
- Do not apply topical medication to the affected area.
- Do not apply any material to the burn.
- Do not apply ice.
- Do not break blisters.

THIRD-DEGREE BURNS

A third-degree burn penetrates the entire thickness of the skin and permanently destroys tissue.

Signs
- Damage to epidermis and all dermis
- Leather-like appearance
- Often painless
- Heals by contracture
- Loss of skin layers
- Skin may appear charred or have patches that appear white, brown, or black

Medical Management for Nurses

Do's

- Cover burn lightly with sterile gauze or clean cloth.
- Take steps to prevent shock: lay the victim flat; elevate the feet about 12 inches.
- Have person sit up if face is burned; watch closely for possible breathing problems.
- In chemical burns, remove or dilute the chemical agent with water.
- Contact the nearest hospital or tertiary medical center that is equipped to handle third-degree burns.

Don'ts

- Do not apply topical medication to the infected area.
- Do not apply any material to the burn.
- Do not apply ice.
- Do not break the blisters.

If the patient has sustained an airway burn and is lying down, do not place a pillow under the victim's head since this procedure can close the airway.

INHALATIONAL INJURY

THERMAL

Thermal damage of the airway is often restricted to the area of the upper airway system. It is caused when heat is dissipated quickly from the dry air to the tissues of the airway once the patient inhales. Steam or very moist hot air has the potential for causing serious injury and deep burns in the trachea and bronchi because the vapor droplets carry a great amount of heat energy. This injury requires immediate medical care and treatment since tissue swelling in the respiratory system may obstruct the airway.

TOXIC

Smoke inhalation is considered to be the leading cause of mortality in burn treatment centers. It results in several conditions, including carbon monoxide and cyanide poisoning. Carbon monoxide (CO) poisoning occurs when CO in the air binds to the cell's hemoglobin with greater affinity than it does to the body's oxygen, thereby decreasing the oxygen-carrying capacity of the red blood cells. Therapy involves providing the patient with high-flow and/or hyperbaric oxygen. Cyanide poisoning results when the combustion of various elements present in the fire (e.g., plastics, fabrics, rubber) forms cyanide compounds, which then act as a cellular asphyxiant and interfere with cellular oxidation through the cytochrome a_3 system. Therapy involves administering a mixture of amyl nitrite, sodium nitrite, and sodium thiosulfate.

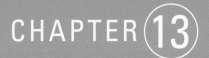

CHAPTER 13

Victim Assessment and Management

CRITICAL INFO

- Tetanus is a potential health threat for persons who sustain wound injuries.
- Expect a variety of infection types because of exposure to various elements of the surrounding environment.
- Provide tetanus prophylaxis to any wounded patient.

OVERVIEW

The risk for sustaining an injury during and following a disaster is high. Tetanus is a potential health threat for persons who sustain wound injuries. Any wound or rash has the potential for becoming infected and should be assessed by a healthcare provider as soon as possible. Quick and proper management of wounds is critical to prevent further problems such as amputations. Nurses should abide by the following basic wound management steps in order to maximize their effectiveness and efficiency in aiding patients.

EVALUATION AND PRETREATMENT CONSIDERATIONS FOR NURSES

- Ensure that the scene is safe for you to approach the patient and that, if necessary, it is secured by the proper authorities before patient evaluation.
- Observe universal precautions while participating in all aspects of wound care.
- Obtain a focused history from the patient, and perform an appropriate examination to exclude additional injuries.
- Be alert for the presence of other injuries in patients with wounds.
- Expect a variety of infection types because of exposure to various elements of the surrounding environment.
- Wounds contaminated by soil can become infected.
- Puncture wounds can carry bits of clothing and debris into the wound, resulting in infection.
- Crush injuries are more susceptible to infection than are wounds from shearing forces.

Victim Assessment and Management

TREATMENT

- Remove constricting rings or other jewelry from the injured body part.
- Apply direct pressure to any bleeding wound to control hemorrhage.
- Examine wounds for gross contamination, devitalized tissue, and foreign bodies.
- Remove devitalized tissue and foreign bodies before repair as they may increase the incidence of infection.
- Cleanse the wound periphery with soap and sterile water or available solutions, and provide anesthetics and analgesia whenever possible.
- Irrigate wounds with saline solution using a large-bore needle and syringe; bottled water is acceptable if no other solution is available.
- Leave contaminated wounds open; wounds that are sutured in an unsterile environment may trap bacteria and are at high risk for infection.
- Clip hair close to the wound; shaving of hair is not necessary and may increase the chance of wound infection.
- Cover wounds with dry dressing; deeper wounds may require packing with saline-soaked gauze and subsequent coverage with a dry bulky dressing.
- Provide tetanus prophylaxis to any wounded patient.

On-Scene Management

CRITICAL INFO

- If the authorities have not yet been alerted, call 911.
- Approach the scene with caution and treat as a crime scene until determined otherwise.
- Be prepared to speak with law enforcement personnel regarding your observations.

OVERVIEW

Each disaster situation is unique. The mental, physical, and emotional strains of experiencing a disaster affect everyone differently and are something for which you cannot prepare. Nurses must possess the ingenuity, flexibility, adaptability, creativity, and understanding of the need to expand their practice parameters beyond those for which they are normally accustomed. All nurses providing care in an emergency situation must be competent in the basic principles of first aid.

MINIMUM CORE COMPETENCIES

See Table 14-1 for minimum core competencies in assessment and therapeutics.

UPON ARRIVAL AT THE SCENE

- Approach with caution.
- Assess the scene by looking, listening, and smelling to ensure your safety.
- Be aware of persons and vehicles around or leaving the scene.
- Remain alert and attentive.
- Treat as a crime scene until determined otherwise (terrorism is a crime; therefore the scene of a potential terrorist release must be treated as a crime scene).
- If the authorities have not yet been alerted, alert them by calling 911.

PREVENTING NURSING CASUALTIES

An injured or infected nurse diminishes the number of those able to provide care and increases those in need of care. The following are important considerations:

TABLE 14-1   Minimum Core Competencies

ASSESSMENTS	THERAPEUTICS
• Perform respiratory, airway assessment. • Perform cardiovascular assessment, including vital signs, monitoring for signs of shock. • Perform integumentary assessment, including burn assessment. • Perform pain assessment. • Perform trauma assessment from head to toe. • Perform mental status assessment including Glasgow coma scale. • Know indications for intubation. • Perform IV insertion and administration of IV medications. • Understand emergency medications. • Understand principles of fluid therapy.	• Concepts of basic first aid • Triage and transport • Pain management • Management of hypovolemia and fluid replacement • Suturing (if appropriate based on practice parameters) and initial wound care • Blast injuries/dealing with tissue loss • Eye lavage techniques • Chemical exposures • Fractures/immobilization of fractures • Crush injuries • Movement of patients with spinal cord injury

On-Scene Management

- Determine if isolation of patients is necessary in the event of a bioterrorist attack.
- Determine if the environment is safe (e.g., structural problems, preserving safety of supplies).
- Determine the need for personal protective equipment in the event of a chemical or radiological event.
- Evacuate casualties and potential casualties first.

ON-SCENE CONSIDERATIONS

- Try not to discard any potential evidence and help prevent other individuals from destroying possible evidence.
- Ensure that proper measures were taken to decontaminate evidence.
- Maintain documentation for all patients and their belongings.
- Ensure that any items belonging to patients are bagged and labeled appropriately (see Chapter 11 if relevant).
- Remove nonauthorized personnel from the scene (e.g., media, politicians, etc.).

- Ensure that the worried-well are not bypassing security and triage measures.
- Be prepared to speak to law enforcement personnel regarding your observations.

ESSENTIAL RESPONSE EQUIPMENT

- Registered nurse license; this will help deter imposters
- Form of identification
- Stethoscope
- Packaged snack
- Bottled water
- Change of clothing

OTHER AGENCY RESPONSIBILITIES

Local enforcement agencies and the FBI will be conducting an investigation of the crime scene while you work to treat and provide care to patients. You should be aware of the fact that these agencies are there to collect evidence as well as to protect you. They may at times call upon you to assist in their investigation; however, for the most part, they will be working around you. Among their responsibilities are the following:

- Identify and establish the perimeters.
- Protect and secure scene boundaries.
- Document actions and observations.
- Control all individuals at the scene.
- Prevent individuals from altering or destroying possible evidence.
- Identify suspects, witnesses, and bystanders.
- Remove nonauthorized personnel from the scene (e.g., media, politicians).
- Ensure that the worried-well are not bypassing security and triage measures.

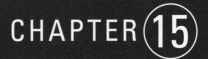

CHAPTER 15

Psychological Considerations

CRITICAL INFO

- Everyone who experiences a disaster is affected by it.
- Most people pull together and function during and after a disaster, but their effectiveness is diminished.
- Disaster stress and grief reactions are normal responses to an abnormal situation.
- Most people do not see themselves as needing mental health services following a disaster and will not seek such services; survivors may reject disaster assistance of all types.
- Use an active outreach approach to intervene successfully in a disaster.
- Survivors respond to active, genuine interest and concern.

OVERVIEW

People who have experienced a disaster are coping with the disruption and loss caused by that disaster. In most instances, these individuals are normal, well-functioning people who do not see themselves as needing mental health services and are thus unlikely to request them. Therefore nurses and mental health workers must play an active role in searching for survivors at churches, senior centers, local cafes, schools, and community centers rather than waiting and expecting survivors to come to them. Nurses should be culturally sensitive, provide information in the languages spoken, and work with local, trusted organizations and community leaders to better understand and assess survivors' needs. This chapter will provide a foundation for those nurses expected to handle the psychological aspect of a disaster.

HUMAN RESPONSES TO DISASTER

It is important to understand that most people who are exposed to disasters do not develop major psychopathology or lifelong psychological problems resulting from their exposure to disaster. In fact, only a small percentage of disaster survivors develop significant psychiatric considerations. Many others, however, will suffer more minor and transient psychological effects.

Disasters produce a range of psychological and psychosocial consequences in their aftermath. When we talk about the psychological impact of disaster, we mean specifically the emotional characteristics and associated behaviors of those individuals affected. When we talk about the psychosocial impact of disaster, we look at how these emotional characteristics and associated behaviors affect individuals' interactions with others and the resulting life challenges they will experience.

For those exposed to disaster, the aftermath can feel like an emotional roller coaster. Many find themselves flooded with various feelings and thoughts that can affect the way they respond and recover from disaster. An individuals' reactions to and recovery from disaster are influenced by a number of factors such as the specific characteristics of the disaster and the community disaster response.

RESPONSES TO NATURAL AND HUMAN-CAUSED DISASTERS

NATURAL DISASTERS

For most natural disasters, the causal agent is seen as beyond human control and without evil intent. (From this perspective, individuals may fare better in coping with natural disasters than they do with disasters that are human-caused, depending on the level of exposure.) Survivors affected by natural disasters typically struggle with property loss and damage, the need to relocate to temporary or permanent housing, the financial stress associated with the loss of possessions or time away from their jobs, and the daily challenges of negotiating with insurance companies and disaster relief agencies. These are valid stressors and ones that should not be minimized when considering the emotional toll on those impacted by such disasters.

We also know, all too well, that natural disasters can result in significant loss of life or injuries. Under these circumstances, the psychological impact may look more like those resulting from human-caused disasters than from natural disasters.

HUMAN-CAUSED DISASTERS

Human-caused disasters, on the other hand, can stem from a number of reasons that for many may seem senseless and incomprehensible, making recovery from such events even more challenging. Whether such actions result from an inherent sense of evil; political, sociological, or religious beliefs; mental illness; or hate or bias against an individual or group, the perception that the event was preventable or avoidable and the sense of betrayal by mankind can produce significant psychological challenges for those exposed to human-caused acts.

Individuals exposed to human-caused disasters are confronted with the reality that bad things can happen to good people. They lose their illusion of invulnerability and realize that anyone can be in the wrong place at the wrong time. Their basic assumptions about humanity may be shattered, and they no longer feel that the world is secure, fair, and orderly. They may

Psychological Considerations

also be faced with the palpable realization that even their government cannot guarantee their safety and protection or that of their family and loved ones.

POPULATION EXPOSURE MODEL

WHO IS AFFECTED BY DISASTERS?

Many educators and researchers who have contributed to the field of disaster mental health have attempted to define and clarify those individuals who are most likely to be affected by disaster. One such approach takes a macro level view of the entire community and the gradations of effects and needs across population groups. This population exposure model is a series of concentric circles depicting the various affected populations following a disaster.

The closer the populations are to the center, the more directly they are impacted by the disaster. However, keep in mind that individuals within these populations may experience a range of responses that fall outside what is expected based on the population's proximity to the disaster. These populations are described in Table 15-1.

TABLE 15-1	Populations Affected by Disaster
DESIGNATION	**POPULATION DESCRIPTION**
Population A	• Community victims killed and seriously injured • Bereaved family members, loved ones, close friends
Population B	• Community victims exposed to the incident and disaster scene, but not injured
Population C	• Bereaved extended family members and friends • Residents in disaster zone whose homes were destroyed • First responders, rescue and recovery workers • Medical examiner's office staff • Service providers immediately involved with bereaved families, obtaining information for body identification and death notification
Population D	• Mental health and crime victim assistance providers • Clergy, chaplains • Emergency healthcare providers • Government officials • Members of media
Population E	• Groups that identify with target-victim group • Businesses with financial impacts • Community-at-large

POST-DISASTER REACTIONS

INDIVIDUAL REACTIONS AND CHARACTERISTICS

Clinicians have struggled with why disaster survivors, when exposed to identical trauma and tragedy, respond with considerable variability. Some individuals are able to incorporate the experience into their lives; others continue to feel devastated and overwhelmed, suffering lasting psychological problems that prevent them from moving on with their lives. In the immediate aftermath of a large-scale disaster, those individuals suffering direct exposure may typically be seen as most at-risk, but other individual characteristics influence how people respond and recover from disaster. Post-trauma reactions are expressed through different pathways: physical, behavioral, emotional, and cognitive (Table 15-2).

TABLE 15-2   Post-Trauma Reactions

EMOTIONAL EFFECTS	COGNITIVE EFFECTS
• Shock • Anger and resentment • Anxiety and fear • Despair and hopelessness • Emotional numbing and apathy • Terror • Guilt • Grief and sadness • Irritability • Helplessness and loss of control • Feelings of insignificance • Loss of interest • Variability in mood ("mood swings")	• Difficulty concentrating and thinking • Difficulty making decisions • Memory impairment and forgetfulness • Disbelief • Confusion • Distortion of sense of time • Decreased self-esteem • Decreased self-efficacy • Self-blame • Intrusive thoughts, memories, and flashbacks • Worry
PHYSICAL EFFECTS	**BEHAVIORAL EFFECTS**
• Fatigue • Insomnia • Sleep disturbance • Agitation • Physical complaints • Headaches • Gastrointestinal problems • Decreased or increased appetite • Decreased or increased sex drive • Exaggerated startle response	• Crying spells • Outbursts and acts of aggression • Social withdrawal and avoidance • Relationship conflict • School and work impairment

Psychological
Considerations

Possible post-disaster reactions include the following:
- A concern for basic survival
- Grief over loss of loved ones and loss of valued and meaningful possessions
- Fear and anxiety about personal safety and the physical safety of loved ones
- Sleep disturbances, often including nightmares and imagery from the disaster
- Concerns about relocation and the related isolation or crowded living conditions
- A need to talk about events and feelings associated with the disaster, often repeatedly
- A need to feel one is a part of the community and its recovery efforts

PSYCHOLOGICAL TRIAGE

Targeting interventions to those at greatest risk is both more efficient and more effective than attempting to provide mental health interventions to everyone who has been exposed. The following characteristics increase the likelihood of psychiatric morbidity and are ranked from most to least likely:

1. Threat to one's life
2. Infliction of physical injuries
3. Exposure to the dead and mutilated
4. Witnessing unexpected and violent death
5. Learning of the unexpected and violent death of a loved one
6. Learning one has been exposed to chemical or biological toxins
7. Causing death or severe harm to another
8. Knowledge that the infliction of pain and suffering was deliberate (such as in the Oklahoma City bombing and the terrorist attacks of September 11, 2001)

PSYCHOLOGICAL FIRST AID

Psychological first aid (PFA) is currently considered as the intervention of choice in the immediate aftermath of a disaster. Although there is no evidence-based literature supporting the efficacy of this intervention at the time of this writing, many components of PFA are based in crisis intervention and stress management approaches.

The concept of psychological first aid is similar to that of medical first aid in that we are trying to sustain life, promote safety and survival, comfort and reassure, and provide protection to those who have experienced a traumatic event. PFA helps people get through the immediate phase of the disaster by building on their existing resources and helping develop a sense of empowerment and safety.

Once exposure to a disaster has already occurred, efforts must then be directed toward the reduction of psychological harm (Tables 15-3 and 15-4).

THE PUBLIC'S REACTION

People who have experienced terrorism or a natural disaster may have a wide range of reactions, but panic is not a common one; more often helpful and adaptive behaviors prevail. Fear should not be misunderstood or mislabeled as panic; it is a normal and often appropriate response to very frightening circumstances. However, the possibility of mass hysteria/panic still exists. Mass hysteria/panic has been referred to as a condition when individuals are consumed by such an enormous fear that their actions are conducted solely in self-interest and, as such, their actions lead to loss of social organization, loss of social roles, and overall chaos. Providing clear and concise information as well as specific tasks may lessen panic and increase the sense of control.

ENVIRONMENTAL EFFECTS
- Civil unrest
- Hoaxes
- Mass suicide

NURSING IMPLICATIONS
- Treating patients with medically unexplained physical symptoms; this may not differ from routine emergency care in that the etiology of symptoms is often unknown.
- Prepare to treat fractures and head injuries that may result from a mass exodus or public panic.

PSYCHOLOGICAL CONDITIONS

ACUTE STRESS DISORDER (ASD)
Acute stress disorder is the disorder most likely to be encountered by the disaster response team.
- Signs and symptoms: anxiety; dissociation
- Onset: within 1 month of trauma
- Duration: minimum of 2 days

Psychological
Considerations

TABLE 15-3   Psychological First Aid Measures

FIRST AID	COMMENT
Remove individuals from ongoing trauma.	If patient is showing signs of acute stress disorder, encourage patient to rest and assist in connecting with available sources of social support.
Educate patients.	Individuals will be comforted by knowing that their reactions are normal after experiencing extreme stress.
Prevent retraumatization.	Limit number of persons with whom victims must interact in order to receive services, and also reduce amount of red tape required.
Prevent new victims.	Limit number of people exposed to sights, sounds, and smells of a disaster site, whenever possible.
Prevent "pathologizing" distress.	Avoid labeling normal reactions as pathological; this can prevent symptoms from being interpreted as a medical condition or disorder that requires treatment.
Allow silence.	Silence gives survivor time to reflect and become aware of feelings; "being with" survivor and his/her experience is very supportive.
Attend nonverbally.	Eye contact, head nodding, and caring facial expressions let survivors know you are in tune with them.
Actively listen.	Repeating portions of what person has said conveys interest, understanding, and empathy; paraphrasing also clarifies meaning and checks for misunderstandings.
Reflect feelings.	If survivor's tone of voice or nonverbal gestures suggest anger, sadness, or fear, the worker may state, "You sound/appear angry, scared, etc.; does that fit for you?" This helps survivor to identify and articulate his/her emotions.
Allow expression of emotions.	Expression of intense emotions through tears or angry venting is an important part of healing; it often helps survivor work through feelings so that he/she can better engage in constructive problem solving; workers should stay relaxed, breathe, and let the survivor know that it is okay to feel these emotions.

TABLE 15-4	Communication Guidelines for Psychological First Aid	
DO SAY		**DON'T SAY**
• These are normal reactions to a disaster. • It is understandable that you feel this way. • You are not going crazy. • It wasn't your fault; you did the best you could. • Things may never be the same, but they will get better, and you will feel better.		• It could have been worse. • You can always get another pet/car/house. • It's best if you just stay busy. • I know just how you feel. • You need to get on with your life.

If symptoms persist longer than 4 weeks' post-trauma, a diagnosis of post-traumatic stress disorder (PTSD) should be considered. For the diagnosis of PTSD to be made, the person should have been exposed to a traumatic event in which both of the following were present:

1. The person experienced, witnessed, or was confronted with an event or events that involved actual or threatened death or serious injury, or a threat to the physical integrity of self or others.
2. The person's response involved intense fear, helplessness, or horror.

Either while experiencing or after experiencing the distressing event, the individual has three (or more) of the following dissociative symptoms:

1. A subjective sense of numbing, detachment, or absence of emotional responsiveness
2. A reduction in awareness of his or her surroundings (e.g., "being in a daze")
3. Derealization
4. Depersonalization
5. Dissociative amnesia (i.e., inability to recall an important aspect of the trauma)

The traumatic event is persistently re-experienced in at least one of the following ways:

- Recurrent images, thoughts, dreams, illusions, flashback episodes, a sense of reliving the experience, or distress from exposure to reminders of the traumatic event
- Marked avoidance of stimuli that arouse recollections of the trauma (e.g., thoughts, feelings, conversations, activities, places, people)
- Marked symptoms of anxiety or increased arousal (e.g., difficulty sleeping, irritability, poor concentration, hypervigilance, exaggerated startle response, motor restlessness)

Psychological Considerations

The disturbance causes clinically significant distress or impairment in social, occupational, or other important areas of functioning or impairs the individual's ability to pursue some necessary task, such as obtaining necessary assistance or mobilizing personal resources by telling family members about the traumatic experience.

The disturbance lasts for a minimum of 2 days and a maximum of 4 weeks and occurs within 4 weeks of the traumatic event.

The disturbance is not due to the direct physiological effects of a substance (e.g., a drug of abuse, a medication) or a general medical condition, is not better accounted for by brief psychotic disorder, and is not merely an exacerbation of a pre-existing disorder.

GENERALIZED ANXIETY DISORDER

Generalized anxiety disorder is excessive anxiety and worry (apprehensive expectation), occurring more days than not for at least 6 months, about a number of events or activities (such as work or school performance).

The anxiety and worry are associated with three (or more) of the following six symptoms (with at least some symptoms present for more days than not for the past 6 months):
- Restlessness or feeling keyed up or on edge
- Being easily fatigued
- Difficulty concentrating or mind going blank
- Irritability
- Muscle tension
- Sleep disturbance (difficulty falling or staying asleep, or restless unsatisfying sleep)

NOTE: Only one symptom is required in children.

The focus of the anxiety and worry is not confined to features of an axis I disorder—for example, the anxiety or worry is not about having a panic attack (as in panic disorder), being embarrassed in public (as in social phobia), being contaminated (as in obsessive-compulsive disorder), being away from home or close relatives (as in separation anxiety disorder), gaining weight (as in anorexia nervosa), having multiple physical complaints (as in somatization disorder), or having a serious illness (as in hypochondriasis)—and the anxiety and worry do not occur exclusively during post-traumatic stress disorder.

The anxiety, worry, or physical symptoms cause clinically significant distress or impairment in social, occupational, or other important areas of functioning.

The disturbance is not due to the direct physiological effects of a substance (e.g., a drug of abuse, a medication) or a general medical condition (e.g., hyperthyroidism) and does not occur exclusively during a mood disorder, a psychotic disorder, or a pervasive developmental disorder.

POST-TRAUMATIC STRESS DISORDER (PTSD)

Post-traumatic stress disorder is an intense physical and emotional response to thoughts and reminders of the event that last for many weeks or months after the traumatic event. Table 15-5 summarizes (by category) the symptoms associated with PTSD. (**NOTE:** The duration of these symptoms must be more than 1 month.)

VICARIOUS TRAUMA (SECONDARY TRAUMA, COMPASSION FATIGUE)

Vicarious trauma is defined as indirect exposure to trauma through a first-hand account of a traumatic event. The vivid recounting of trauma by the survivor and the clinician's emotional response may result in a type of post-traumatic stress disorder characterized by nightmares, intrusive thoughts, depression, anxiety, burnout, or desensitization (Table 15-6).

TABLE 15-5	PTSD Symptoms by Category
CATEGORY	**SYMPTOMS**
Reliving	• Flashbacks • Nightmares • Feeling guilty • Extreme fear of harm • Numbing of emotions • Uncontrollable shaking • Chills or heart palpitations • Tension headaches
Avoidance	• Staying away from activities, places, thoughts, or feelings related to the trauma • Feeling detached or estranged from others
Increased arousal	• Being overly alert or easily startled • Difficulty sleeping • Irritability or outbursts of anger • Lack of concentration
Other	• Panic attacks • Depression • Suicidal thoughts and feelings • Drug abuse • Feelings of being estranged and isolated • Not being able to complete daily tasks

Psychological Considerations

TABLE 15-6 Vicarious Trauma	
ISSUES AND CONCERNS	**NURSING RESPONSE**
• Physical and psychological effects of work overload and exposure to human suffering • Experience physical stress symptoms • Become increasingly irritable • Depressed • Overinvolved or unproductive • Show cognitive effects such as difficulty concentrating or making decisions	• Establish a clear chain of command and reporting relationships. • Establish shifts no longer than 12 hours with 12 hours off. • Clearly define intervention goals and strategies appropriate to assignment setting. • Establish a buddy system for support and monitoring stress reactions. • Have a positive atmosphere of support and tolerance with "good job" said often. • Assess workers' functioning regularly. • Rotate workers between low-, mid-, and high-stress tasks. • Encourage breaks and time away from assignment. • Educate about signs and symptoms of worker stress and coping strategies. • Provide individual and group defusing and debriefing. • Encourage physical exercise and muscle stretching. • Encourage nutritious eating. • Maintain contact of primary social supports. • Reduce physical tension by taking deep breaths, calming self through meditation, and walking mindfully. • Talk about emotions and reactions with co-workers.

Psychological
Considerations

CONFIDENTIALITY

A helping person is in a privileged position. Helping a survivor in need infers a sharing of problems, concerns, and anxieties—sometimes with intimate details. This special sharing cannot be done without a sense of trust, built upon mutual respect, and the explicit understanding that all discussions are confidential and private. No case should be discussed elsewhere without the consent of the person being helped (except in an extreme emergency when it is judged that the person will harm himself or others). It is only by maintaining the trust and respect of the survivor that the privilege of helping can continue to be exercised.

MENTAL HEALTH REFERRALS

Referrals to a mental health professional ought to be made when one or more of the symptoms in Table 15-7 are present.

TABLE 15-7	Symptom List for Referral to a Mental Health Professional
Disorientation	• Dazed • Memory loss • Inability to give date or time, state where he or she is, recall events of past 24 hours, or understand what is happening
Depression	• Pervasive feelings of hopelessness and despair • Unshakable feelings of worthlessness and inadequacy • Withdrawal from others • Inability to engage in productive activity
Anxiety	• Constantly on-edge • Restless • Agitated • Inability to sleep • Frightening nightmares • Flashbacks and intrusive thoughts • Obsessive fears of another disaster • Excessive ruminations about the disaster
Mental illness	• Hearing voices • Seeing visions • Delusional thinking • Excessive preoccupation with an idea or thought • Pronounced pressure of speech (e.g., talking rapidly with limited content continuity)
Inability to care for self	• Not eating, bathing, or changing clothes • Inability to manage activities of daily living
Suicidal or homicidal thoughts or plans	• Excessive thinking or talking of death • Thinking of inflicting harm
Problematic use of alcohol or drugs	• Constantly thinking or talking about drinking alcohol or taking drugs • Using alcohol or drugs more than "normal" • Hiding alcohol or drugs • Not eating
Domestic violence, child abuse, or elder abuse	• Restless • Agitated • Short temper • Urge to hit

Psychological Considerations

POTENTIAL RISK GROUPS

Each community affected by a disaster has its own demographic composition, cultural representation, and prior experience with disasters and thus has a different reaction to the traumatic events. The following groups are particularly vulnerable to coping with a disaster and should be given special consideration:

- Age groups
- Cultural and ethnic groups
- People with serious and persistent mental illness
- People in group facilities
- Human service and disaster relief workers

AGE GROUPS

Each age group is vulnerable in unique ways to the stresses of a disaster and should be treated differently. Disaster stress reactions appear at different times following an emergency, and it is important for mental health workers to be familiar with the possible manifestations of psychological trauma.

Table 15-8 describes possible disaster reactions of the different age groups and helpful responses to them.

CULTURAL AND ETHNIC GROUPS

Table 15-9 describes possible issues and concerns related to culture and ethnicity, as well as appropriate nursing responses.

PEOPLE WITH SERIOUS AND PERSISTENT MENTAL ILLNESS

Many disaster survivors with mental illness function fairly well following a disaster, if most essential services have not been interrupted. They have the same capacity to "rise to the occasion" and perform as heroically as the general population during the immediate aftermath of the disaster. However, for others who may have achieved only a tenuous balance before the disaster, additional mental health support services, medications, or hospitalization may be necessary to regain stability. For survivors diagnosed with PTSD, disaster stimuli (e.g., helicopters, sirens) may trigger an exacerbation caused by associations with prior traumatic events.

The range of disaster mental health services designed for the general population is equally beneficial for survivors with mental illness; disaster stress affects all groups. Workers need to be aware of how people with mental illness are perceiving disaster assistance and services and build bridges that facilitate access where necessary.

TABLE 15-8	Disaster Reactions by Age and Nursing Responses	
AGE	**ISSUES AND CONCERNS**	**NURSING RESPONSE**
1-5	• Resumption of bed-wetting, thumb-sucking, clinging to parents • Fears of the dark • Avoidance of sleeping alone • Increased crying • Loss of appetite • Stomach aches • Nausea • Sleep problems, nightmares • Speech difficulties • Tics • Anxiety, fear • Irritability, angry outbursts • Sadness, withdrawal	• Give verbal assurance and physical comfort. • Provide comforting bedtime routines. • Avoid unnecessary separations. • Permit child to sleep in parents' room temporarily. • Encourage expression regarding losses (e.g., deaths, pets, toys). • Monitor media exposure to disaster trauma. • Encourage expression through play activities.
6-11	• Decline in school performance • Aggressive behavior at home or school • Hyperactive or silly behavior • Whining, clinging, acting like a younger child • Increased competition with younger siblings for parents' attention • Change in appetite • Headaches • Stomach aches • Sleep disturbances, nightmares • School avoidance • Withdrawal from friends, familiar activities • Angry outbursts • Obsessive preoccupation with death	• Give additional attention and consideration. • Relax expectations of performance at home and at school temporarily. • Set gentle but firm limits for acting-out behavior. • Provide structured but undemanding home chores and rehabilitation activities. • Encourage verbal and play expression of thoughts and feelings. • Listen to child's repeated retelling of a disaster event. • Involve child in preparation of family emergency kit, home drills. • Rehearse safety measures for future disasters. • Coordinate school disaster program for peer support, expressive activities, education on disasters, preparedness planning, identifying at-risk children.
12-18	• Decline in academic performance • Rebellion at home or school • Decline in previous responsible behavior	• Give additional attention and consideration. • Relax expectations of performance at home and school temporarily.

Psychological Considerations

Continued

TABLE 15-8	Disaster Reactions by Age and Nursing Responses—cont'd	
AGE	**ISSUES AND CONCERNS**	**NURSING RESPONSE**
12-18	• Agitation or decrease in energy level, apathy • Delinquent behavior • Social withdrawal • Appetite changes • Headaches • Gastrointestinal problems • Skin eruptions • Complaints of vague aches and pains • Sleep disorders • Loss of interest in peer social activities, hobbies, recreation • Sadness or depression • Resistance to authority • Feelings of inadequacy and helplessness	• Encourage discussion of disaster experiences with peers, significant adults. • Avoid insistence on discussion of feelings with parents. • Encourage physical activities. • Rehearse family safety measures for future disasters. • Encourage resumption of social activities, athletics, clubs, etc. • Encourage participation in community rehabilitation and reclamation work. • Coordinate school programs for peer support and debriefing, preparedness planning, volunteer community recovery, identifying at-risk teens.
Adults	• Sleep problems • Avoidance of reminders • Excessive activity level • Crying easily • Increased conflicts with family • Hypervigilance • Isolation, withdrawal • Fatigue, exhaustion • Gastrointestinal distress • Appetite change • Somatic complaints • Worsening of chronic conditions • Depression, sadness • Irritability, anger • Anxiety, fear • Despair, hopelessness • Guilt, self-doubt • Mood swings	• Provide supportive listening and opportunity to talk in detail about disaster experiences. • Assist with prioritizing and problem solving. • Offer assistance for family members to facilitate communication and effective functioning. • Assess and refer when indicated. • Provide information on disaster stress and coping, children's reactions, and families. • Provide information on referral resources.
Older adults	• Withdrawal and isolation • Reluctance to leave home • Mobility limitations • Relocation adjustment problems	• Provide strong and persistent verbal reassurance. • Provide orienting information. • Use multiple assessment methods, as problems may be under-reported.

| TABLE 15-8 | Disaster Reactions by Age and Nursing Responses—cont'd | |

AGE	ISSUES AND CONCERNS	NURSING RESPONSE
Older adults	• Worsening of chronic illnesses • Sleep disorders • Memory problems • Somatic symptoms • More susceptible to hypothermia and hyperthermia • Physical and sensory limitations (sight, hearing) interfere with recovery • Depression, despair about losses • Apathy • Confusion, disorientation • Suspicion • Agitation, anger • Fears of institutionalization • Anxiety with unfamiliar surroundings • Embarrassment about receiving "hand outs"	• Provide assistance with recovery of possessions. • Assist in obtaining medical and financial assistance. • Assist in reestablishing familial and social contacts. • Give special attention to suitable residential relocation. • Encourage discussion of disaster losses and expression of emotions. • Provide and facilitate referrals for disaster assistance. • Engage providers of transportation, chore services, meal programs, home health, and home visits as needed.

| TABLE 15-9 | Culture and Ethnicity in Disaster Response |

ISSUES AND CONCERNS	NURSING RESPONSE
• Socioeconomic conditions • Language barriers • Suspicion of governmental programs because of prior experiences • Rejection of outside interference or assistance • Differing cultural values	• Be culturally sensitive; information and application procedures should be translated into primary spoken languages and available in nonwritten forms. • Learn about cultural norms, traditions, local history, and community politics from leaders and social service workers indigenous to groups being served. • Establishing working relationships with trusted organizations, service providers, and community leaders often facilitates increased acceptance. • Be respectful and well-informed, and dependably follow through on stated plans.

Psychological Considerations

TABLE 15-10 Disaster Response for People in Group Facilities

ISSUES AND CONCERNS	NURSING RESPONSE
• Anxiety • Panic • Frustration as a consequence of limited mobility and dependence on caretakers • Fear of evacuation and relocation • Dependence on others for care or on medical resources for survival contributes to heightened fear and anxiety • Change in physical surroundings, caregiving personnel, and routines can be extremely difficult	• Reestablish familiar routines. • Provide supportive opportunities to talk about disaster experiences. • Assist with making contact with loved ones. • Provide information on reactions to disaster and coping.

PEOPLE IN GROUP FACILITIES

Table 15-10 describes possible issues and concerns related to people in group facilities, as well as appropriate nursing responses.

Psychological
Considerations

Disaster Settings

CRITICAL INFO

- Nurses working in shelters must assess the needs of the shelter population and provide 24-hour health coverage for the residents.

OVERVIEW

Nurses provide care in many settings before, during, or after a disaster occurs. Frequently, it is an American Red Cross established shelter. Service centers are often opened after the disaster, but healthcare, first aid, and procurement of needed goods and equipment are provided in the shelter before service centers open. The following list provides other types of settings associated with the provision of disaster care:

- Emergency aid stations
- Emergency operations center (EOC)
- Family assistance centers (FACs)
- Home or hospital visits
- Outreach
- Phone banks and hotlines
- Points of dispensing (POD) centers
- Respite centers
- Reunification/family reception center
- Service centers
- Shelter
- Staging areas
- Temporary morgue

EMERGENCY AID STATIONS

Emergency aid stations are rapid-response, temporary, mobile or stationary units, often located in the heart of the disaster area. Emergency aid station teams frequently consist of a physician or emergency medical services (EMS) provider, a nurse, a case worker, and a mental health worker. Stabilization and basic first aid are provided, and triage and transportation to other healthcare facilities is arranged.

EMERGENCY OPERATIONS CENTER

Ongoing mental health support services may also be requested at the emergency operations center (EOC). In the aftermath of a large-scale disaster, the EOC is a chaotic and stressful environment as county and other organizational disaster planners and managers are preparing the disaster relief response.

Disaster Settings

FAMILY ASSISTANCE CENTERS

Family assistance centers (FACs) are commonly opened in the event of a disaster involving mass casualties or fatalities. These centers usually offer a range of services in an effort to meet the needs of individuals under these circumstances. Mental health services, spiritual care, mass care (feeding), and crime victims' services, as well as the services of law enforcement, the medical examiner, disaster relief agencies, and other local, state, and federal agencies, are also offered on-site. Family assistance centers are usually located away from the immediate disaster site, though it is important to note that many times family members will request visits to the affected site or memorial services will be planned, and thus the FAC should be close enough to facilitate those activities.

HOME OR HOSPITAL VISITS

Visits are made to the home or hospital to provide assistance if a person(s) cannot come to a service center. Nurses evaluate living conditions, determine healthcare assistance needed, or provide support when a death is disaster related (condolence call).

OUTREACH

Similar to a home visit, the purpose of outreach is to meet victims/individuals in the affected area, provide needed goods and services, and make community assessments. Disaster response teams may be dispersed in communities to reach individuals who have not been able to come to a shelter or service center.

People evacuate to many places during a disaster, often to other cities. They may not be able to immediately return to their home or reach a service center.

PHONE BANKS AND HOTLINES

Communities may wish to set up a phone bank to address and respond to numerous questions that typically arise regarding the availability of disaster relief services and resources after a large-scale disaster. These phone banks are likely to be overwhelmed in the first few hours or days with many questions or concerns regarding such issues as locating missing family members, providing information on shelter or mass food distribution sites, or answering healthcare concerns or issues.

POINTS OF DISPENSING (POD) CENTERS

Points of dispensing centers might be established by local, state, or federal public health agencies in the event of a public health emergency. These centers may be established to provide mass distribution of medications or vaccinations in an effort to prevent or mitigate the spread of any communicable disease or other public health risk.

RESPITE CENTERS

Respite centers are locations where first responders can rest and obtain food and clothing and other basic support services. The decision to open a respite center is usually determined if there is evidence that prolonged rescue and recovery efforts are necessary. Respite centers are usually located in close proximity to the direct impact of a disaster.

REUNIFICATION/FAMILY RECEPTION CENTERS

This may be located near the site of a disaster such as civil violence, an aviation incident, or other disaster when family members are separated.

Family reception centers are typically opened in the immediate aftermath of a disaster involving mass casualties or fatalities. There is a common recognition that after such disasters, individuals may be trying to locate family or other loved ones specifically involved in the disaster or estranged during the evacuation process. Often these are temporary holding sites until a more structured and operational family assistance center can be opened. Family reception centers may be established in close proximity to the immediate disaster scene where individuals arrive in search of family and other loved ones involved in the incident.

SERVICE CENTERS

A service center is a central location to provide health services and information and referral to those affected by the disaster. The service center may be located within the shelter facility or other location that is convenient to the community at large.

Nurses may be asked to provide health services and assessments at a service center. They may be asked to help maintain safe, sanitary conditions at the service center in addition to providing emergency or urgent healthcare needs.

Service centers may be opened by a local or federal governmental agency or by disaster relief organizations to meet the initial needs of disaster survivors. These centers typically offer assistance with locating temporary housing or providing for the immediate personal needs of disaster survivors, such as food, clothing, and clean-up materials.

SHELTER

A shelter is temporary, short-term emergency housing for people affected or threatened by a disaster. Most commonly, the American Red Cross local chapters establish partnerships in the community with churches, schools,

Disaster
Settings

and other facilities to provide shelter for the immediate needs of the community. Immediate needs are food, water, shelter, and security.

Nurses working in shelters must assess the needs of the shelter population and provide 24-hour health coverage for the residents. Those victims who are ill and/or injured should be referred to community health facilities or local healthcare professionals, and those with immediate first aid needs should receive care in the shelter. Disaster victims may need replacement of medications or equipment such as crutches or wheel chairs. The nurse is a member of the shelter response team and should collaborate with the shelter manager and local resources for medication and other vital equipment needed in a shelter.

Additional nursing responsibilities in the shelter are providing patient/ victim education, being aware of proper disposal of needles (used by people with diabetes, arthritis, or multiple sclerosis, for example), recognizing biohazard materials, assisting victims with any special dietary needs, and maintaining a sanitary environment at the shelter.

STAGING AREAS

A staging area may be established as close as possible to an area expecting the impact of a disaster so first responders and other healthcare workers can be deployed to the disaster site quickly.

In the event of large-scale disasters requiring significant volunteer resources, a volunteer staging area may be established by a particular disaster relief agency or by a local, state, or federal government agency. Typically, activities in the volunteer staging area include the registering of volunteers for duty and the credentialing of those involved in duties requiring specific skill sets such as mental health or health services. It is important for you to understand that you will be assigned to a service site where you are needed most. While you may have a preference for one site over another, the response needs will require you to be flexible. Survivors or relief personnel are equally important in response to mental health.

TEMPORARY MORGUE

Nurses are vital members of the team when a temporary morgue is established. A temporary morgue is established following large-scale disasters such as the September 11 terrorist attacks or the Oklahoma City bombing. Assessing and providing care for family members and friends are a critical post-disaster nursing activity.

Disaster Settings

COMMON SHELTER NURSING RESPONSIBILITIES

QUESTIONS TO ASK

- How did your illness or injury occur?
- When did your illness or injury occur?
- Was the illness or injury caused or aggravated by the disaster?
- Do you have any healthcare insurance, Medicaid, or Medicare?
- Is follow-up care needed (doctor visit, physical therapy, etc.)?
- Are any bandages, medical equipment, or prescriptions needed?

Advocacy

- Encourage victims to remain active participants in decision-making.
- Reassure victims that they will handle the situation adequately.
- Assist the victim in making health appointments for follow-up.
- Explore options for donations or reduced fees for prescriptions.
- Use in-kind donations if available for bandages.

Eyeglasses or Contact Lenses

- Do you have optical insurance?
- What is the name of your eye doctor?
- Where is he located?
- When was your last eye examination?
- Do you have a spare pair of glasses?
- If contacts were lost, do you have eyeglasses with the same prescription?

Dentures or Partial Bridge

- What happened to your dentures?
- Do you have insurance?
- What is the name of your dentist?
- Where is he located?
- When did you get your dentures or partial?

Prosthetic Devices or Durable Medical Equipment

- What happened to your crutches, wheel chair, or prosthesis?
- Did the disaster create a need to have this equipment?
- When and where was it obtained?
- Do you have insurance to cover the cost of the item?
- What is the name and address of the supplier?
- Do you need it temporarily or permanently?
- Can it be repaired?

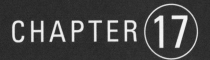

Mass Immunization Clinics

> ## CRITICAL INFO
>
> - To determine vaccine-specific contraindications, event specifications, and vaccine specifications, contact the CDC's National Immunization Program at 1-800-CDC-INFO or NIPINFO@cdc.gov.

OVERVIEW

In the event of a disaster, clinics may need to be established in order to accommodate the large number of patients who will require vaccination and/or prophylactic treatment. These clinics will allow nurses to quickly and efficiently direct patients from the prescreening process all the way through the immunization process. Nurses will play a critical role in the administration of the clinic and will serve in a variety of functions such as nurse clinic manager, nurse practitioner, medical screener, and immunizer.

CLINIC SITE INFORMATION

Sites that can be used for clinics in the event of an emergency are non-hospital locations where vaccine and/or prophylactic medications could be administered to a large number of exposed or potentially exposed patients. Since clinic sites will need to host hundreds, and possibly thousands, of patients, they are primarily selected based on their capacity [(clients/hour) = (# of nurses) × (20-60 clients/hour)]. Schools are thus often a preferred location because of their size and physical structure (e.g., parking lots, long corridors, large classrooms, cafeterias, private offices) as well as the availability of resources such as tables, chairs, and restrooms. Enclosed sports' arenas and other facilities at local universities can also serve as clinic sites. Local employers may also choose to set up sites to vaccinate staff and family members.

Recently some public health departments have instituted an alternative "drive through" vaccination model that has proved to be successful. In a nondisaster situation, this model eliminates barriers such as parking, appointments, standing in long lines, and inclement weather. There are three nursing roles in the drive through model: screening, drawing, and administering the vaccine. It may be necessary to use local law enforcement to direct traffic.

PRIORITIES FOR VACCINATION/ PROPHYLACTIC MEDICATION

See Table 17-1 for priority levels for administration of vaccinations and prophylactic medication.

IMMUNIZATION AND PROPHYLAXIS CLINIC FLOW

There are nine clinic stations, and descriptions of each station follow:
1. Prescreening
2. Initial screening
3. Triage station
4. Interpretation station
5. Registration and sign-in station
6. Prophylactic/vaccine medication preparation area

TABLE 17-1	Priorities for Vaccinations and Prophylactic Medications	
PRIORITY	**GROUP**	**DESCRIPTION**
1	Distribution personnel	Healthcare workers and public health personnel involved in distribution of vaccine/ prophylactic medication
	Personnel involved in direct contact with patients	Involved in evaluation, care, or transportation of confirmed, probable, or suspected patients
	Laboratory personnel	Involved in collecting or processing clinical specimens from confirmed, probable, or suspected patients
	Persons responsible for community safety and security	Police and firefighters
	Groups likely to be exposed to infectious materials	Laundry workers and medical waste handlers
	Highly skilled persons who provide essential community services	Nuclear power plant, telecommunications, and electrical grid operators
	Persons exposed to initial release	Friends, family, or relatives
2	Face-to-face contacts of cases	

Mass Immunization Clinics

7. Prophylaxis/vaccination station
8. Pregnant station
9. Problem station

PRESCREENING

- Observe clients as they arrive at the clinic to screen for obvious signs of illness.
- Follow standard precautions in accordance with emergency medical services (EMS) and Hazmat guidelines.
- Direct those with illness and symptoms immediately to the sick station.

INITIAL SCREENING

- Establish eligibility to receive vaccine/prophylactic medication.
- Review address identification, referrals, or any information needed to determine eligibility.

TRIAGE STATION

- Separate and direct clients to the appropriate station according to the following:
  - Those who are pregnant go to the pregnant station.
  - Those who are "well" go to the interpretation station.
  - Those with documentation of previous prophylaxis/vaccination are referred out of the receiving line to the problem station.
- Distribute information statements to those receiving vaccine/prophylactic medication.

INTERPRETATION STATION

All clients who are "well" should receive vaccine/prophylactic medication and be referred to this station for the following:

- Conduct counseling and review of the most current information statements; two-way verbal communication is essential to obtain informed consent, especially with non–English-speaking individuals.
- Ask females about pregnancy status or suspected pregnancy; if a positive response is received about pregnancy status, refer client to the pregnant station.
- Discuss precautions and contraindications before administration, according to the latest CDC recommendations.
- Refer clients to the next registration and sign-in station.

REGISTRATION AND SIGN-IN STATION

Verify client information at this station:
- Verify personal information and record date of information statements.
- This list may be used for consent of prophylaxis/vaccination if clinic policies have this requirement.
- After obtaining signature and verifying information from client, refer to the prophylaxis/vaccination station.
- Sign-in sheet should include patient information (e.g., name, birthday, address, phone number), clinic information (e.g., name, address, contact person, contact number, county), and vaccine information (e.g., date, lot number, vaccine check).

PROPHYLACTIC/VACCINE MEDICATION PREPARATION AREA

- Staff prepares vaccine for administration.
- Staff repackages medications into individual doses/quantities.
- Supply manager or pharmacy manager maintains centralized inventory of vaccine/prophylactic medication.

PROPHYLAXIS/VACCINATION STATION

Clients receive prophylaxis/vaccination at this station; the clinician takes the following actions:
- Ensure counseling was given to client before administering vaccine/prophylactic medication.
- Give documentation of vaccine/prophylactic medication.
- Give instructions regarding importance of completing medication or returning for additional doses of vaccine; inform patients of tracking/recall procedures.
- Make available standing orders and an emergency kit for possible reactions to vaccine/first dose of medication.

PREGNANT STATION

- Determine name of prenatal provider
- Provide necessary counseling regarding vaccine-specific contraindications during pregnancy.

PROBLEM STATION

Those with documentation of previous prophylaxis/vaccination or clients who have a history of or current symptoms of illness (e.g., rash or obvious signs of illness) should be referred to the problem station for evaluation by a physician or nurse practitioner (NP).

Mass Immunization Clinics

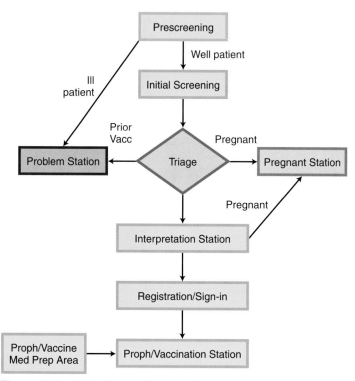

Figure 17-1. Typical mass immunization clinic stations and patient flow.

- If indicated, transport clients with rash illness to nearest care facility, with the least exposure to other clients.
- Fill out case investigation form.

Figure 17-1 shows a patient flow chart that demonstrates how patients will be directed between the stations.

Legal Implications

CRITICAL INFO

- Healthcare laws vary by state—to obtain the most accurate information for your specific state, please check with your healthcare organization.
- For states that have ratified the Model State Emergency Health Powers Act (MSEPHA), once a public health emergency is declared, the Governor has the ability to order in-state doctors, nurses, pharmacists, and all other medical personnel to treat people.
- Certain states have implemented Good Samaritan laws, which limit the liability of medical professionals when they render care in an emergency situation.

OVERVIEW

Law refers to the rules and regulations under which nurses must carry out their professional duties. Laws can come from many different sources, including statutes, regulations, and decisions of the appellate courts. All of these sources of law can affect nurses in many different ways. For example, laws may require nurses to perform some affirmative act, such as report new cases of certain diseases to the local or state health department. There may be criminal penalties for those who fail to comply with these requirements. The laws may also give the authority to certain government officers to require nurses to either do or refrain from doing something in a particular circumstance. Law can also create certain responsibilities for nurses, such as laws that impose civil liability for the failure to provide professionally adequate care. Nursing professionals should be familiar with the written rules and regulations when questions arise concerning the proper course of conduct in a disaster situation.

STATE POLICE POWERS

A state has the authority and responsibility to protect the public's health from threats resulting from a natural outbreak of an infectious disease as well as from intentional acts of terrorism. This authority is derived from its inherent "police powers" and is granted to the states through the Tenth Amendment. As a result of exercising its police powers, the state government has the authority to enact laws and promote regulations to safeguard the health, safety, and welfare of its citizens.

Among these laws and regulations is the authority to invoke isolation and quarantine, mandate vaccination, require healthcare providers to report and collect new cases of diseases, and compel treatment for contagious diseases such as tuberculosis. In 2002 the Model State Emergency Health Powers Act (MSEHPA) was enacted in several states to further strengthen public health infrastructure. MSEHPA has the following five basic functions:

1. Preparedness
2. Surveillance
3. Management of healthcare supplies to ensure adequate supplies
4. Powers to compel vaccination, testing, treatment, isolation, and quarantine when necessary
5. Communication, providing clear and authoritative information to the public

REPORTING TO WORK

For states that have ratified MSEPHA, once a public health emergency is declared, the Governor has the ability to order in-state doctors, nurses, pharmacists, and all other medical personnel to treat people. Providers may be required to assist in the performance of vaccination, treatment, examination, or testing of any individual as a condition of licensure, authorization, or the ability to continue to function as a healthcare provider in the state. Healthcare providers from out-of-state may also be called upon to assist in response efforts.

LIABILITY

Certain states have implemented Good Samaritan laws, which limit the liability of medical professionals when they render care in emergency situations.

ISOLATION AND QUARANTINE

Isolation refers to the separation of persons who have a specific infectious illness from those who are healthy and the restriction of their movement to stop the spread of that illness. Quarantine refers to the separation and restriction of movement of persons who, while not yet ill, have been exposed to an infectious agent and therefore may become infectious. Both isolation and quarantine are public health strategies that have proven effective in stopping the spread of infectious diseases.

Legal Implications

CDC QUARANTINE AUTHORITY

Title 42 U.S. Code Section 264 (Section 361 of the Public Health Service [PHS] Act) gives the Secretary of Health and Human Services (HHS) responsibility for preventing the introduction, transmission, and spread of communicable diseases from foreign countries into the United States and within the United States and its territories/possessions. This statute is implemented through regulations found at 42 CFR Parts 70 and 71. Under its delegated authority, the CDC is empowered to detain, medically examine, or conditionally release individuals reasonably believed to be carrying a communicable disease.

CDC INTENT TO USE QUARANTINE POWERS

In general, the CDC defers to the state and local health authorities in their primary use of their own separate quarantine powers. Based upon long experience and collaborative working relationships with our state and local partners, the CDC continues to anticipate the need to use this federal authority to quarantine an exposed person only in rare situations, such as events at ports of entry or in similar time-sensitive settings.

QUARANTINABLE INFECTIOUS DISEASES

Federal law further stipulates that isolation and quarantine are mandated for certain communicable diseases through executive order of the President. The following communicable diseases are included:
- Cholera
- Diphtheria
- Infectious tuberculosis
- Plague
- Smallpox
- Yellow fever
- Viral hemorrhagic fevers (Lassa, Marburg, Ebola, Crimean-Congo, South American, and others)
- Severe acute respiratory syndrome (SARS)
- Novel or re-emergent influenza viruses that may cause a pandemic

VACCINATION

States have the authority to compel vaccination, even when an individual refuses to comply with mandatory vaccination laws.

TREATMENT

Most state public health laws mandate treatment of such contagious diseases as sexually transmitted diseases or tuberculosis. For other contagious diseases, people should be given the option of undergoing treatment or entering voluntary isolation or quarantine.

PATIENT PRIVACY

Despite Health Insurance Portability and Accountability Act (HIPAA) regulations, two provisions exist that may allow healthcare providers to have access to patient-protected information (45 CFR 164.512[b]). Patient privacy may be circumvented when the protected information is disseminated to public health authorities "for public health activities and purposes," or when medical information is used for the purposes of public health surveillance, investigation, or intervention (HIPAA, 2003).

YOUR STATE'S LAWS

Complete Table 18-1 with your state's information.

TABLE 18-1 Your State's Laws Relating to Nursing Disaster	
LAW, STATUTE, OR REGULATIONS	**YOUR STATE**
Can my state mandate medical exams and tests?	
Can my state mandate the vaccination and treatment of individuals against their wishes?	
Can my state enforce isolation and quarantine?	
Can my state grant access to protected health information to public health and medical authorities?	
Can my state require me to report to work?	
Can my state protect me against civil liability?	

Legal
Implications

APPENDIX

Ⓐ

FAMILY DISASTER PLAN

OVERVIEW

One of the most important steps you can take in preparing for emergencies is to develop a household disaster plan. This involves creating a plan that identifies who you can contact in an emergency, what each member of your family must do, and how you can better prepare yourself for the situation.

Use the sections below as a guide in creating your family disaster plan and ensuring that you are prepared to respond in the event of a disaster.

YOUR FAMILY'S DISASTER PLAN

Learn about the natural disasters that could occur in your community and learn how you can respond to them.

Possible hazards in my area:
1.
2.
3.
4.
5.
6.
7.
8.

Post emergency phone numbers next to all telephones.
Police department:
Fire department:
Local emergency services:
Healthcare provider(s):
Local emergency management office:
Local American Red Cross:
Poison Help: 1-800-222-1222

Other important names and numbers:
_____
_____
_____

Talk with employers and school officials about their emergency response plans.
Name of school:
Address:
Phone:

Prepare a family communication plan so that each member of the family can contact one another.

NAME	ADDRESS	EMAIL	PHONE #

CHILD	DAYCARE/SCHOOL	PHONE #

Identify two meeting places for your household in the event you are separated.

The first should be near your home and the second should be away from your area in case you cannot return home.

Name of place #1:

Address:

Phone:

Name of place #2:

Address:

Phone:

Pick a friend or relative who lives out of the area for household members to call to say they are okay.

Make sure everyone has a cell phone, calling card, or coins to make the phone call. Teach young children how to call long distance.

Name of contact:

Phone:

Email:

Make sure everyone in your household knows how and when to shut off water, gas, and electricity at the main switches; consult with your local utilities if you have questions.

Name of local utilities company:

Phone:

Have transportation and evacuation plans ready.

Make sure you have an extra tank of gas since gas stations may be closed or overwhelmed. If you do not have a car, make plans with a neighbor or your local government to be evacuated.

Contact person/agency:

Address:

Phone:

Stay up to date with all of your certifications (e.g., CPR, ACLS, PALS, TNCC).

Certification #1:

Date of completion/renewal:

Certification #2:

Date of completion/renewal:

Certification #3:

Date of completion/renewal:

Reduce the economic impact of disaster on your property and your household members' health and financial well-being.

- Review property insurance policies before disaster strikes—make sure policies are current and be certain they meet your needs (type of coverage, amount of coverage, and hazard covered—flood, earthquake).
- Protect your household's financial well-being before a disaster strikes—review life insurance policies and consider saving money in an "emergency" savings account that could be used in any crisis. It is advisable to keep a small amount of cash or traveler's checks at home in a safe place where you can quickly gain access to it in case of an evacuation.
- Be certain that health insurance policies are current and meet the needs of your household.

Keep important documents safe and in a watertight container.

Make sure you have copies of important documents as well.

IMPORTANT ITEMS	PLACE OF STORAGE
Personal identification	
Cash and coins	
Credit cards	
Extra set of house keys and car keys	

Continued

IMPORTANT ITEMS	PLACE OF STORAGE
Copies of the following:	
Birth certificate	
Marriage certificate	
Driver's license	
Social Security cards	
Passports	
Wills	
Deeds	
Inventory of household goods	
Insurance papers	
Immunization records	
Bank and credit card account numbers	
Stocks and bonds	
Emergency contact list and phone numbers	
Map of the area and phone numbers of places you could go	

Consider ways to help neighbors who may need special assistance, such as the elderly or the disabled.

NAME	SPECIAL NEED	ADDRESS	PHONE #

Make arrangements for pets.
Pets are not allowed in public shelters. Service animals for those who depend on them are allowed.

Name of veterinarian:
Address:
Phone:
Name of animal shelter:
Address:
Phone:

Draw a floor plan of your home; mark two escape routes from each room.

Keep an emergency money supply.

People with special needs:
If you or someone in your family has a disability or special need, you may have to take these additional steps to protect yourself and your household in an emergency:

1. Find out about special assistance that may be available in your community. Register with the office of emergency services or fire department for assistance, so needed help can be provided quickly in an emergency.
2. Create a network of neighbors, relatives, friends, and co-workers to aid you in an emergency.
3. Discuss your needs with your employer.
4. If you are mobility-impaired and live or work in a high-rise building, have an escape chair.
5. If you live in an apartment building, ask the management to mark accessible exits clearly and to make arrangements to help you evacuate the building.
6. Keep extra wheelchair batteries, oxygen, catheters, medication, food for guide or hearing-ear dogs, or other items you might need.
7. Those who are not disabled should learn who in their neighborhood or building is disabled so that they may assist them during emergencies.
8. If you are a caregiver for a person with special needs, make sure you have a plan to communicate if an emergency occurs.

DISASTER SUPPLY KITS

You and your family may need to survive on your own for 3 days or more. You should prepare emergency supplies for the following situations:

- A disaster supply kit with essential food, water, and supplies for at least 3 days—this kit should be kept in a designated place and be ready to "grab and go" in case you have to leave your home quickly because of a disaster, such as a flash flood or major chemical emergency. Make sure all household members know where the kit is kept.
- Consider having additional supplies for sheltering or home confinement for up to 2 weeks.
- You should also have a disaster supply kit at work. This should be in one container, ready to "grab and go" in case you have to evacuate the building.

• A car kit of emergency supplies, including food and water, to keep stored in your car at all times. This kit would also include flares, jumper cables, and seasonal supplies.

Water: The Absolute Necessity

1. Stocking water reserves should be a top priority. Drinking water in emergency situations should not be rationed. Therefore it is critical to store adequate amounts of water for your household.
   • Individual needs vary, depending on age, physical condition, activity, diet, and climate. A normally active person needs at least 2 quarts of water daily just for drinking. Children, nursing mothers, and ill people need more. Very hot temperatures can double the amount of water needed.
   • Since you will also need water for sanitary purposes and, possibly, for cooking, you should store at least 1 gallon of water per person per day.
2. Store water in thoroughly washed plastic, fiberglass, or enamel-lined metal containers. Do not use containers that can break, such as glass bottles.
   • Containers for water should be rinsed with a diluted bleach solution (1 part bleach to 10 parts water) before use. Previously used bottles or other containers may be contaminated with microbes or chemicals. Do not rely on untested devices for decontaminating water.
   • If your water is treated commercially by a water utility, you do not need to treat water before storing it. Additional treatments of treated public water will not increase storage life.
   • If you have a well or public water that has not been treated, follow the treatment instructions provided by your public health service or water provider.
   • If you suspect that your well may be contaminated, contact your local or state health department or agriculture extension agent for specific advice.
   • Seal your water containers tightly, label them, and store them in a cool, dark place.
   • It is important to change stored water every 6 months.

Food: Preparing an Emergency Supply

1. If activity is reduced, healthy people can survive on half their usual food intake for an extended period or without any food for many days. Food, unlike water, may be rationed safely, except for children and pregnant women.

2. You do not need to go out and buy unfamiliar foods to prepare an emergency food supply. You can use the canned foods, dry mixes, and other staples on your cupboard shelves. Canned foods do not require cooking, water, or special preparation. Be sure to include a manual can opener.

3. Keep canned foods in a dry place where the temperature is fairly cool. To protect boxed foods from pests and to extend their shelf life, store the food in tightly closed plastic or metal containers.

4. Replace items in your food supply every 6 months. Throw out any canned good that becomes swollen, dented, or corroded. Use foods before they go bad, and replace them with fresh supplies. Date each food item with a marker. Place new items at the back of the storage area and older ones in front.

5. Food items that you might consider including in your disaster supply kit include the following: ready-to-eat meats, fruits, and vegetables; canned or boxed juices, milk, and soup; high-energy foods such as peanut butter, jelly, low-sodium crackers, granola bars, and trail mix; vitamins; foods for infants or persons on special diets; cookies, hard candy; instant coffee, cereals, and powdered milk.

First Aid Supplies

Assemble a first aid kit for your home and for each vehicle.

1. The basics for your first aid kit should include the following items:
   - First aid manual
   - Sterile adhesive bandages in assorted sizes
   - Assorted sizes of safety pins
   - Cleansing agents
   - Antibiotic ointment
   - Latex gloves (2 pairs)
   - Petroleum jelly or other lubricant
   - 2-inch and 4-inch sterile gauze pads (4-6 of each size)
   - Triangular bandages (3)
   - Sunscreen
   - Scissors
   - 2-inch and 3-inch sterile roller bandages (3 rolls each)
   - Cotton balls
   - Tweezers
   - Needle
   - Moistened towelettes
   - Antiseptic
   - Thermometer
   - Tongue depressor blades (2)

2. Ask your physician or pharmacist about storing prescription medications. Be sure they are stored to meet instructions on the label and be mindful of expiration dates—be sure to keep your stored medication up to date.
3. Have an extra pair of prescription glasses or contact lenses.
4. Have the following nonprescription drugs in your disaster supply kit:
   - Aspirin and non-aspirin pain relievers
   - Antidiarrhea medication
   - Antacid (for stomach upset)
   - Laxative
   - Vitamins
   - Syrup of ipecac

Tools and Emergency Supplies

It will be important to assemble these items in a disaster supply kit in case you have to leave your home quickly.

1. Tools and other items:
   - A portable, battery-powered radio, TV, and alarm clock
   - Flashlight and extra batteries
   - Signal flare
   - Matches in a waterproof container
   - Shut-off wrench, pliers, shovel, and other tools
   - Duct tape and scissors
   - Plastic sheeting
   - Whistle
   - A-B-C–type fire extinguisher
   - Tube tent
   - Compass
   - Work gloves
   - Paper, pens, and pencils
   - Needles and thread
2. Sanitation and hygiene items:
   - Washcloth and towel
   - Towelettes, soap, hand sanitizer, liquid detergent
   - Toiletries
   - Heavy-duty plastic garbage bags
   - Medium-sized plastic bucket with tight lid, small shovel for digging a latrine
   - Disinfectant and household chlorine bleach
3. Kitchen items:
   - Manual can opener
   - Mess kits or paper cups, plates, and plastic utensils

- All-purpose knife
- Household liquid bleach to treat drinking water (⅛ teaspoon of unscented Clorox bleach per gallon of water)
- Sugar, salt, pepper
- Aluminum foil and plastic wrap
- Re-sealing plastic bags
- If food must be cooked, small cooking stove and a can of cooking fuel

4. Household documents and contact numbers:
   - Personal identification, cash, traveler's checks, or credit card
   - Copies of important documents
   - Emergency contact list and phone numbers
   - Map of the area and phone numbers of place you could go
   - An extra set of car keys and house keys

Clothes and Bedding

- One complete change of clothing and footwear for each household member. Shoes should be sturdy work shoes or boots. Also include rain gear, hat and gloves, extra socks, extra underwear, thermal underwear, sunglasses.
- Blankets or a sleeping bag for each household member, pillows.

Specialty Items

Remember to consider the needs of infants, elderly persons, disabled persons, and pets and to include entertainment and comfort items for children.
- For baby
- For the elderly
- For pets
- Entertainment: books, games, quiet toys, and stuffed animals

HEALTHCARE STAFF PREPAREDNESS

In an emergency situation, your healthcare facility may be required to assist in the care and treatment of a potentially large number of patients. All employees of the facility should be prepared to respond. Effective preparedness should include disaster training and practice drills.

GENERAL TRAINING

General training would provide nurses with the basic knowledge and skills needed to respond to a disaster emergency. Some of the following topics are addressed in training programs:
1. Basic health and safety training
2. Details about CBRNE agents

3. How to use a facility's notification system
4. Different types of PPE and when to use them

PRACTICE DRILLS

Practice drills offer a way for healthcare facilities to test their disaster preparedness plans. Further, The Joint Commission (TJC) requires that healthcare facilities conduct two practice drills a year to maintain their accreditation status.

YOUR FACILITY'S DISASTER TRAINING

Date(s) of my training:
Date(s) of practice drills(s):
Topics covered in your training session:

PERSONAL STRENGTHS AND WEAKNESSES

_____
_____

YOUR ROLE IN A DISASTER

Where I must report:
To whom I must report:
My responsibilities: _____
_____
_____
_____

PERSONAL PROTECTIVE EQUIPMENT

In an emergency, wearing the proper PPE can be critical to remaining safe and staying alive. You should be familiar with the different levels of PPE and how to use them.

YOUR PPE CHECKLIST

In a CBRNE event, I would be expected to decontaminate *patients:*
Yes
No
In a CBRNE event, I would be expected to decontaminate the *facility:*
Yes
No
I have training in the following PPE:
Date(s) of training:
Location of PPE:
Who to contact in case PPE requires maintenance:

APPENDIX

B

CONTACTS: LOCAL AND STATE PUBLIC HEALTH INFORMATION

OVERVIEW

This section is intended for your use to list state and local contact information. Phone numbers for federal agencies can be found at the end of this appendix.

LOCAL AND STATE PUBLIC HEALTH CONTACTS

Local Department of Health
Name:
Address:
City, State, Zip:
Phone:
Fax:
Email:

State Department of Health
Name:
Address:
City, State, Zip:
Phone:
Fax:
Email:

FEDERAL AGENCY CONTACT INFORMATION

AGENCY	PHONE	NOTES
American Burn Association	1-800-548-2876	
Armed Forces Radiobiology Research Institute, Medical Radiobiology Team	1-301-295-0530	
CDC Emergency Response Hotline	1-707-488-7100	
CDC National Immunization Program	1-800-CDC-INFO	NIPINFO@cdc.gov
National Center for Injury Prevention and Control	1-770-488-1506	

AGENCY	PHONE	NOTES
Radiation Emergency Assistance Center/Training Site (REAC/TS)	1-865-576-3131	M-F 8 AM to 4:30 PM EST or 1-865-576-1005 after hours

OTHER IMPORTANT NUMBERS

Add other important numbers below.

Appendix B

GLOSSARY OF TERMS AND ACRONYMS

ABCDEs Airway, breathing, circulation and control, disability, expose, and environment

ABCs Airway, breathing, and circulation

ABG Arterial blood gas

ACCOLC Access overload control (for cellular radio telephones)

ADFAA Aviation Disaster Family Assistance Act of 1996

ANFO Ammonium nitrate fuel oil

ANSI American National Standard for Personal Protection

ARC American Red Cross

ARDS Acute respiratory distress syndrome

ARS Acute radiation syndrome

ASD Acute stress disorder

Assets A term used for all resources required, including human, to adequately respond to a disaster

ATSDR Agency for Toxic Substances Disease Registry

Bioterrorism The unlawful release of biological agents or toxins with the intent to intimidate or coerce a government or civilian population to further political or social objectives; humans, animals, and plants are often targets

BSE Bovine spongiform encephalopathy

BSS Burn size score

Case One (unit) documented incidence of disease

Casualty Any person suffering physical and/or psychological damage that leads to death, injury, or material loss

CBRNE Chemical, biological, radiological, nuclear, and explosive events

CDC Centers for Disease Control and Prevention

CJD Creutzfeldt-Jakob disease

CNS Central nervous system

CO Carbon monoxide

Contamination An accidental release of hazardous chemicals or nuclear materials that pollute the environment and place humans at risk of contamination

Contingency plan An emergency plan developed in expectation of a disaster; often based on hazard identification and risk assessment, the availability of human and material resources, and overall community preparedness

COPD Chronic obstructive pulmonary disease

Covert release (of a biological agent) An unannounced release of a biological agent that causes illness; if undetected, a covert release of the contagion has the potential to spread widely before it is detected

CPR Cardiopulmonary resuscitation

CRI Cutaneous radiation injury

Crisis management Administrative measures that identify, acquire, and plan for the resources needed to anticipate, prevent, and/or resolve a threat to public health and safety

CV Cardiovascular

Decontamination The removal of hazardous chemicals or nuclear substances from the skin and/or mucous membranes by showering or washing the affected area with water, or by rinsing with a sterile solution

Disaster Any event, typically occurring suddenly, that causes damage, ecological disruption, loss of human life, deterioration of health and health services, AND that exceeds the capacity of the affected community on a scale sufficient to require outside assistance—these events can be caused by nature, equipment malfunction, human error, or biological hazards and disease (e.g., earthquake, flood, fire, hurricane, cyclone, typhoon, significant storms, volcanic eruptions, spills, air crashes, drought, epidemic, food shortages, civil strife)

Disaster continuum The life cycle of a disaster or emergency

Disaster paradigm Organizes the provider's preparation and response to disaster management into eight steps (**D,** detect; **I,** incident command; **S,** scene safety and security; **A,** assess hazards; **S,** support; **T,** triage and treatment; **E,** evacuation; and **R,** recovery)

DTPA Diethylenetriaminepentaacetate

Economic impact Catastrophic disasters, depending upon the type, scope, and magnitude of the disaster incident, could threaten the economic sustainability of the communities affected and may cause severe disruption and long-term economic damage. Extreme disaster incidents can generate cascading economic situations extending outside the immediate community. Even in moderate disasters, of all businesses that close following a disaster, more than 43% never reopen, and an additional 29% close permanently within 2 years

ED Emergency department

EEE Eastern equine encephalitis

EID Emerging infectious disease

ELISA Enzyme-linked immunosorbent assay

EMA Emergency Management Agency

Emergency Any natural or manmade situation that results in severe injury, harm, or loss of humans or property

Emergency Management Agency (EMA) Also referred to as the Office of Emergency Preparedness (OEP), the EMA, under the authority of the governor's office, coordinates the efforts of the state's health department, housing and social service agencies, and public safety agencies (e.g., state police) during an emergency or disaster; the EMA also coordinates federal resources made available to the states, such as the National Guard, the Centers for Disease Control (e.g., Epidemic Intelligence Service [EIS] officers), and the Public Health Service (e.g., Agency for Toxic Substances Disease Registry [ATSDR])

Emergency medical services (EMS) system The coordination of the prehospital system (e.g., public access, dispatch, EMTs and medics, ambulance services) and the in-hospital system (e.g., emergency departments, hospitals, and other definitive care facilities and personnel) to provide emergency medical care

Emergency operations center (EOC) The site from which civil government officials (e.g., municipal, county, state, federal) direct emergency operations in a disaster

Emergency support function (ESF) A functional area of response activity established to coordinate the delivery of federal assistance during the response phase of an emergency (ESF's mission is to save lives, protect property, preserve public health, and maintain public safety; ESF represents the type of federal assistance most needed by states overwhelmed by the impact of a catastrophic event on local and state resources)

EMS Emergency medical services

EMT Emergency medical technician

Environmental impact Catastrophic natural and manmade disasters and terrorist attacks can result in extreme environmental impacts that challenge government and community recovery time. Long after the emergency phase subsides, contamination from disasters may remain, consisting of chemical, biological, or radiological materials. While decontamination technologies may be well established for some types of contamination, others are only moderately effective—some contaminants, especially radionuclides, are very difficult and costly to remediate. While some decontamination techniques may be effective in small sites, these techniques may not be suited for decontaminating expansive areas of varying physical characteristics. Evacuation and relocation during cleanup and restoration activities can result in significant business loss and failure, leading to local and regional economic downturn. In addition, agricultural and industrial products from an area contaminated, or thought to be contaminated, can generate impacts that extend within a region and beyond

EOC Emergency operations center

EOP Emergency operations plan

Epidemic The occurrence of any known or suspected contagion that occurs in clear excess of normal expectancy (a threatened epidemic occurs when the circumstances are such that a disease may reasonably be anticipated to occur in excess of normal expectancy)

EPR Emergency Preparedness and Response

ESF Emergency support function

ESF 6 Mass Care Mass Care includes sheltering and feeding victims of disaster, providing emergency first aid, reuniting families, and distributing emergency relief supplies; FEMA is designated by the National Response Plan as the primary agency responsible for ESF Mass Care with the American Red Cross acting as a support agency

ESF 8 Health and Medical Lead by the U.S. Public Health Service's Agency for Preparedness and Response (APER), ESF 8 Health and Medical serves as the basis for federal response to the health needs of disaster victims

ESLI End-of-service-life-indicator

Evacuation An organized removal of civilians from a dangerous or potentially dangerous area

Evaluation A detailed review of a disaster relief program designed to determine whether program objectives were met, to assess the program's impact on the community, and to generate "lessons learned" for the design of future projects (evaluations are most often conducted at the completion of important milestones, or at the end of a specified period)

FAC Family assistance center

Federal Emergency Management Agency (FEMA) An independent agency of the U.S. government that provides a single point of accountability for all federal emergency preparedness and mitigation and response activities

FEMA Federal Emergency Management Agency

FFP Fresh frozen plasma

First responder Local police, fire, and emergency medical personnel who arrive first on the scene of an incident and take action to save lives, protect property, and meet basic human needs

GI Gastrointestinal

Gy Gray

HE High-order explosives

HEPA filter High efficiency particulate air filter

HHS Health and Human Services

HICS Hospital Incident Command System

IAP Incident action plan

IC Incident commander

ICRC International Committee of the Red Cross

ICS Incident Command System

IDLH Immediately dangerous to life and health

IFA Immunofluorescence antibody

Impact phase A phase during a disaster where emergency management activities focus on warning and preparedness

Incident action plan (IAP) A written document, developed by the incident commander or the planning section of the ICS, that details which actions will be conducted by the ICS in response to an incident (IAPs are developed for a specific time period, often referred to as operational periods, and are based on the specific needs of an incident. The incident commander is responsible for the oversight and implementation of the IAP)

Incident Command System (ICS) The model for the command, control, and coordination of a response to an emergency; provides the means to coordinate the efforts of individual agencies:

- *Branch*—an organizational level that has functional or geographic responsibility for major parts of the ICS or incident operations. The incident commander may establish geographic branches to resolve span-of-control issues or functional branches to manage specific functions (e.g., law enforcement, fire and emergency medical); a branch is managed by the branch director

- *Division*—the organizational level that has responsibility for operations within a defined geographic area (the division level is the organizational level between single resources, task forces, or strike teams and the branch level)

- *Emergency operations center (EOC)*—the location where department heads, government officials, and volunteer agencies coordinate the response to an emergency

- *Group*—the organizational level that has responsibility for a specified functional assignment in an emergency or disaster (e.g., perimeter control, evacuation, fire suppression, etc.; a group is managed by a group supervisor)

- *Integrated communications*—a system that uses a common communications plan, standard operating procedures, clear text, common frequencies, and common terminology

- *Resource management*—a management style that maximizes the use of and control over assets; this management style reduces the need for unnecessary communications, provides for strict accountability, and ensures the safety of personnel

- *Size-up/assessment*—the identification of a problem and the assessment of the potential consequences (Initially, a size-up is the responsibility of the first officer to arrive at the scene of an emergency. Size-ups continue throughout the response phase and continuously update the status of the incident, evaluate the hazards present, determine the size of the affected area as well as whether the area can be isolated. A size-up also determines if a staging area will be needed and where it should be located to allow for the best flow of personnel and equipment)

- *Span of control*—the number of individuals managed by a single supervisor (the manageable span of control for one supervisor ranges from between three and seven individuals, with five as optimum)

- *Staging area*—an area where resources are kept while awaiting assignment

- *Strike team*—a group of resources of the same size and type (e.g., five patrol units, three drug K-9 teams)

- *Task force*—a combination of single resources that is assembled for a particular operational need with common communications and one leader
- *Top-down*—a command function that is established by the first officer to arrive on the scene, who then becomes the incident commander
- *Unity of command*—a hierarchical methodology that states that each person within an organization should report to only one superior

Intensity A Roman numerical index from I to XII that describes the physical effects of an earthquake to a specific area (These values are subjective. Intensity is a measurement of the nature and spatial extent of the distribution of damage. The most commonly used scale in the 12-point Modified Mercalli Intensity [MMI]. An earthquake has many intensities [perceived effects], but only one magnitude [force]. The MMI does not indicate an earthquake's magnitude)

JAS Job action sheets

JCAHO Joint Commission on Accreditation of Healthcare Organizations **(now referred to as the Joint Commission [TJC])**

LD50 The amount of a substance (the lethal dose) that results in the death of 50% of the subjects who are exposed to it

LE Low-order explosives

Local government A country, city, village, town, district, political subdivision of any state, Indian tribe or authorized tribal organization, or Alaskan native village or organization, including rural communities, unincorporated towns and villages, or any other public entity

LRCS League of the Red Cross and Red Crescent Societies

MAC-ELISA Immunoglobulin M (IgM) antibody-capture enzyme-linked immunosorbent assay

Magnitude A numerical quantity invented by Charles F. Richter that determines the size and scope of an earthquake by using a measure called a Richter (The magnitude of an earthquake is the total amount of energy released after adjusting for differences in epicentral distance and focal depth. Magnitude is determined on the basis of instrumental records, whereas intensity is determined by subjective observations of an earthquake's damage. Moderate earthquakes have magnitudes of 5.5 to 6.9; larger earthquakes have magnitudes of 7.0 to 7.9; and strong earthquakes have magnitudes of 8.0 and greater. The energy of an earthquake increases exponentially with magnitude. For example, a magnitude of 6.0 earthquake releases 31.5 times more energy than a magnitude 5.0 earthquake or approximately 1000 times more energy than a magnitude 4.0 earthquake)

MCE Mass Casualty Event

MCI Mass Casualty Incident

Mitigation Measures taken to reduce the harmful effects of a disaster by attempting to limit the disaster's impact on human health and economic infrastructure

MMI Modified Mercalli Intensity

MSEHPA Model State Emergency Health Powers Act

MSHA Mine Safety and Health Administration

Multiple disaster/terrorist events There is a possibility that multiple disaster or terrorist incidents will occur simultaneously or sequentially. When scoping resource requirements, organizations should always consider the need to respond to multiple incidents of the same type and multiple incidents of different types, at either the same or other geographic locations. These incidents will invariably require the coordination and cooperation of homeland security response organizations across multiple regional, state, and local jurisdictions

National Planning Scenarios The Federal Interagency—coordinated by the Homeland Security Council (HSC) and in partnership with the Department of Homeland Security (DHS)—has developed 15 all-hazards planning scenarios for use in national, federal, state, and local homeland security preparedness activities. These scenarios are designed to be the foundational structure for the development of national preparedness standards from which homeland security capabilities can be measured because they represent threats or hazards of national significance with high consequence

National Response Plan (NRP) The NRP is designed to address the consequences of any disaster or emergency situation in which there is need for federal assistance under the authorities of the Robert T. Stafford Disaster Relief and Emergency Assistance Act, 42 U.S.C. 5121 et seq. Adopted by the federal government in December 2004, the NRP is an all-hazards plan that establishes a single, comprehensive framework for managing domestic incidents across all levels of government and across a spectrum of activities that include prevention, preparedness, response, and recovery. It provides the structure and mechanisms for coordinating federal support to state and local incident managers and for exercising federal authorities and responsibilities incorporating the NIMS structure. The NRP is also the federal government's plan of action when assisting affected states and local jurisdictions in the event of a severe disaster or emergency. The plan consists of 15 emergency support functions (ESFs) and its annexes

Natural disasters Natural phenomena with acute onset and profound effects (e.g., earthquakes, floods, cyclones, tornadoes)

NBC Nuclear/biological/chemical

NIMS National Incident Management System

NIOSH National Institute for Occupational Safety and Health

NRP National Response Plan

NTSB National Transportation Safety Board

OEP Office of Emergency Preparedness

OSHA Occupational Safety and Health Administration

PAPR Powered air purifying respirator

PCR Polymerase chain reaction

PDA Preliminary damage assessment

PFA Psychological first aid

Phases of the emergency planning model The model is composed of five phases, each corresponding to a type of activity involved in preparing for and responding to a disaster; the phases include planning (preparedness), mitigation, response, recovery, and evaluation

PHS Public Health Service

PKEMRA Post Katrina Emergency Management Response Act

Planning To work cooperatively with others in advance of a disaster in order to initiate prevention and preparedness activities

POD centers Points of dispensing centers

Postimpact phase The period of time after a disaster event; often associated with the activities of response and recovery

PPE Personal protective equipment

Preimpact phase The period of time before a disaster strikes; often associated with mitigation and prevention activities

Preparedness All measures and policies taken before an event occurs that allow for prevention, mitigation, and readiness (Preparedness includes designing warning systems, planning for evacuation and relocation, storing food and water, building temporary shelter, devising management strategies, and holding disaster drills and exercises. Contingency planning is also included in preparedness as well as planning for postimpact response and recovery)

Prevention Primary, secondary, and tertiary efforts that help avert an emergency; these activities are commonly referred to as "mitigation" in the emergency management model (for example, prevention activities include cloud seeding to stimulate rain in a fire; in public health terms, prevention refers to actions that prevent the onset or deterioration of disease, disability, and injury)

PRNT Plaque-reduction neutralization test

PTSD Post-traumatic stress disorder

Public health surveillance The systematic collection, analysis, and interpretation of the health data that are used to plan, implement, and evaluate public health programs; also used to determine the need for public health action

rad Radiation absorbed dose

Radiation Energy emitted by atoms that are unstable—radiation with enough energy to create ion pairs in matter

Radioactive contamination The presence of radiation-emitting substances (radioactive materials) in a place where it is not desired

Recovery Actions of responders, government, and the victims that help return an affected community to normal by stimulating community cohesiveness and government involvement (One type of recovery involves repairing infrastructure, damaged buildings, and critical facilities. The recovery period falls between the onset of the emergency and the reconstruction period)

Red Cross (also known as the American Red Cross, or the International Red Cross) A comprehensive designation used for all or one of the components of the International Red Cross and Red Crescent Movement, a worldwide organization active in humanitarian work (This organization has three components: The International Committee of the Red Cross [ICRC], which acts primarily as a neutral intermediary during armed conflict, and includes the Guardian of the Geneva Conventions, an advocate for the protection of war victims; the League of the Red Cross and Red Crescent Societies [LRCS], an international federation of the National Societies, active in nonconflict disasters and natural calamities; and the National Red Cross or Red Crescent Society, a worldwide relief organization specific to individual countries)

Relief Action focused on saving lives (Relief activities often include search and rescue missions, first aid, and restoration of emergency communications and transportation systems. Relief also includes attention to the immediate care of survivors by providing food, clothing, medical treatment, and emotional care)

REMOVE Remove, elevate, motion, ongoing, vascular, exams, and escharotomy

Resource management A management style that maximizes the use of and control over assets; this management style reduces the need for unnecessary communications, provides for strict accountability, and ensures the safety of personnel

Response The phase in a disaster when relief, recovery, and rehabilitation occur; also includes the delivery of services, the management of activities and programs designed to address the immediate and short-term effects of an emergency or disaster

SAR Supplied-air respirator

SARS Severe acute respiratory syndrome

SARS-CoV SARS-associated coronavirus

SCBA Self-contained breathing apparatus

SEB Staphylococcal enterotoxin B

SEMO State Emergency Management Office

Staging area An area where resources are kept while awaiting assignment

START Simple triage and rapid treatment system

Stockpile An area or storehouse where medicine and other supplies are kept in the event of an emergency

Surveillance The ongoing and systematic collection, analysis, and interpretation of health data essential to the planning, implementation, and evaluation of public health practice; systems are designed to disseminate data in a timely manner and often include both data collection and disease monitoring

Table-top exercise Method of evaluation of a disaster preparedness plan

TBSA Total body surface area

TJC The Joint Commission (formerly called Joint Commission on Accreditation of Healthcare Organizations [JCAHO])

Toxin A substance capable of causing a harmful effect

vCJD Variant form of Creutzfeldt-Jakob disease

VEE Venezuelan equine encephalitis

VHFs Viral hemorrhagic fevers

Weapons of mass destruction Any device, material, or substance used in a manner, in a quantity or type, or under circumstances evidencing an intent to cause death or serious injury to persons or significant damage to property

WEE Western equine encephalitis

WHO World Health Organization

WMD Weapons of mass destruction

WNF West Nile fever

REFERENCES

American Burn Association Board of Trustees and the Committee on Organization and Delivery of Burn Care: Disaster management and the ABA Plan, *Journal of Burn Care and Rehabilitation, 26*(2), 102-106, 2005.

American Red Cross: American Red Cross Disaster Services. Available at http://www.redcross.org.

Andrews GA, Auxier JA, Lushbaugh CC: The importance of dosimetry to the medical management of persons exposed to high levels of radiation. In *Personal dosimetry for radiation accidents,* Vienna, 1965, International Atomic Energy Agency.

Benson M, Koenig KL, Schultz CH: Disaster triage: START, then SAVE—a new method of dynamic triage for victims of a catastrophic earthquake, *Prehospital Disaster Med* 11(2):117-124, 1996.

Centers for Disease Control and Prevention (CDC): Update: investigation of bioterrorism-related anthrax and interim guidelines for exposure management and antimicrobial therapy, October 2001, *MMWR* 50(42):909-919, 2001.

Centers for Disease Control and Prevention (CDC): *Mass casualties: burns.* Available at http://www.bt.cdc.gov/masscasualties/burns.asp

Centers for Disease Control and Prevention (CDC): *Smallpox vaccination clinic guide.* Available at http://www.bt.cdc.gov/agent/smallpox/vaccination/pdf/smallpox-vax-clinic-guide.pdf.

Centers for Disease Control and Prevention (CDC): *West Nile virus: clinical description.* Accessed at http://www.cdc.gov/ncidod/dvbid/westnile/clinicians/clindesc.htm.

Gamelli RL: Guidelines for the operation of burn centers, *Journal of Burn Care & Research, 28*(1):133, 2007.

Health Insurance Portability and Accountability Act (HIPAA): *HIPAA Privacy Rule: disclosures for emergency preparedness—a decision tool.* Available at http://www.hhs.gov/ocr/hipaa/decisiontool/.

Health Insurance Portability and Accountability Act (HIPAA): *Medical privacy: national standards to protect the privacy of personal health information.* Available at http://www.hhs.gov/ocr/hipaa/.

Health Insurance Portability and Accountability Act (HIPAA): *Summary of the HIPAA Privacy Rule,* 2003. Available at http://www.hhs.gov/ocr/privacysummary.pdf.

Lechat, MF: Disasters and public health. *Bulletin of the World Health Organization, 57*(1), 11–17, 1979.

Mayer T, Bersoff-Matcha S, Murphy C et al: Inhalational anthrax: clinical presentation of inhalational anthrax following bioterrorism exposure, *JAMA* 286:2549-2553, 2001.

Morens DM, Folkers GK, Fauci AS: The challenge of emerging and re-emerging infectious diseases, *Nature* 430(6996):242-249, 2004.

NIOSH/OSHA/USCG/EPA: *Occupational Safety and Health guidance manual for hazardous waste site activities,* Washington, DC, 1985, Department of Health and Human Services.

Saffle JR, Gibran N, Jordan, M: Defining the ratio of outcomes to resources for triage of burn patients in mass casualties. *Journal of Burn Care & Rehabilitation,* 26(6):478-482, 2005.

Sever MS, Vanholder R, Lameire N: Management of crush-related injuries after disasters, *New Engl J Med* 354:10, 2006.

U.S. Department of Homeland Security: *National Response Framework.* Available at http://www.fema.gov/pdf/emergency/nrf/nrf-core.pdf.

Veenema TG: *Disaster nursing and emergency preparedness for chemical, biological and radiological terrorism and other hazards,* New York, 2003, Springer.

Weinstein RS, Alibek K: *Biological and chemical terrorism: a guide for healthcare providers and first responders,* New York, 2003, p 61, Thieme Medical Publishers.

World Health Organization (WHO): *WHO infection control guidelines for transmissible spongiform encephalopathies. Report of a WHO consultation, Geneva, Switzerland, 23-26 March, 1999.* Available at http://www.who.int/csr/resources/publications/bse/WHO_CDS_CSR_APH_2000_3/en.

World Health Organization. Available at http://www.who.int/en/.

INDEX

A

Abrin, 80
Acute localized melioidosis, 125–126
Acute radiation syndrome (ARS)
  cause of, 158
  classes of, 158
  exposures that cause, 159
  family safety concerns for, 161
  mortality of, 159
  personal safety concerns for, 160
  precautions for, 161
  signs and symptoms of, 159t–160t
  treatment of, 160
Acute respiratory distress syndrome
  (ARDS)
  and avian influenza (bird flu), 50
  and staphylococcal enterotoxin B
    (SEB), 139
Acute stress disorder (ASD)
  duration of, 229, 232
  impairments caused by, 232
  onset of, 229
  and post-traumatic stress disorder
    (PTSD), 231
  and reexperience of traumatic event, 231
  signs and symptoms of, 229, 231
Agency for Toxic Substances and Disease
  Registry (ATSDR), 100
Air purifying respirators, 175
  advantage and disadvantages of, 179t
Airborne precautions, 45–46, 182
  for biological agents, 104–105, 104t
American Association of Poison Control
  Centers (AAPCC), 100

American Burn Association, 209b
  contact information for, 270
American College of Medical
  Toxicology, 100
American Red Cross (ARC)
  and Aviation Disaster Family Assistance
    Act of 1996, 24
  Congressional, Charter, 22–23
  fundamental principles of, 22
  key points to remember about the, 23
  at the local level, 23
  mission of, 22
  service centers establish by, 242
  at the state and the national levels, 23
Ammonia, appearance and odor of, 95t
Andrews lymphocyte nomogram, 160f
Annual seasonal influenza, 45
Anthrax
  cutaneous. *See* Cutaneous anthrax.
  description of, 106–107
  gastrointestinal. *See* Gastrointestinal
    anthrax.
  inhalational. *See* Inhalational anthrax.
Antibiotics, 102
Anxiety, symptoms of, 235t
ARDS. *See* Acute respiratory distress
  syndrome (ARDS).
Arenaviruses, diseases caused by, 147
Argentine hemorrhagic fever. *See* Viral
  hemorrhagic fevers (VHFs).
Armed Forces Radiobiology Research
  Institute, Medical Radiobiology
  Team, 154
  contact information for, 270–271

Page numbers followed by *b* indicate box(es); *f,* figure(s); *t,* table(s).